PILL POPPING

How to get clear

Pill popping

How to get clear

Valerie Curran
and
Susan Golombok

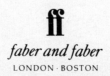

faber and faber
LONDON · BOSTON

Originally published in the UK
under the title of *Bottling It Up*.

Published in the USA by
Faber & Faber, Inc,
39 Thompson Street
Winchester, MA 01890

Library of Congress Cataloging in Publication Data
Curran, Val.
Pill popping.
1. Medication abuse—Social aspects.   2. Tranquilizing
drugs—Social aspects.   3. Women—Mental health.
I. Golombok, Susan.   II. Title.
RM146.5.C87   1985   616.86′3   85–6864
ISBN 0–571–13508–0 (pbk.)

to our mothers

Contents

7

Acknowledgements

Our first and warmest thanks go to all the women who shared their experiences with us and whose voices helped write this book. To the doctors, who gave so generously of their time to discuss the issues we raise, a thousand thanks.

The continued support and advice we received from our professor, Malcolm Lader, and from our colleague and friend, Dr Anna Higgitt, were invaluable and we are very grateful to them both. Thanks also to Philip Tata for his constructive comments and suggestions about the self-help withdrawal programme; to the alternative practitioners for giving so much time to explaining their approaches; to Joan and Marion and the others involved in the self-help groups we visited; to the drug company executives for discussing their viewpoints with us; to Jo for her superb word-processing.

Several friends encouraged us and read earlier drafts of this book – thank you Jan, Jane, Julia, Lisa, Rita, Robin, Padmal and Sue. John Rust, Howard Reid, Amie, Leila, Diane and Mark lived with *Pill Popping* for over a year – very special thanks for your tolerance and support.

Frances Coady was the ultimate in editors, thanks for all your hard work and indestructible humour.

1 Introduction

Everyone knows someone who is bottling it up: people who take pills for their nerves, pills to help them sleep, pills to lift depression or pills to calm them down. Tranquillisers, sleeping pills and antidepressants are offered as chemical solutions to anxiety, insomnia and depression. So many people are using these drugs that Valium, Mogadon, Ativan, Dalmane and Serepax have become international bestsellers and household names.

About a quarter of a million people in Britain[1] and one million in the United States[2] are thought to be addicted to tranquillisers or sleeping pills. One in five women will take these drugs in any one year.[3]

Since the 1980s, when doctors admitted the addictiveness of these drugs, the media have sensationalised the 'Valium Scandal' with headlines proclaiming 'The Dangers of Tranquillity', 'Valiumania', 'The Tranquilliser Trap', 'The Happy Pill can be a Peril', 'The Treachery of the Tranquilliser'. More often than not, this melodramatic treatment of such a serious issue has not only angered the medical profession but also frightened people who take tranquillisers and sleeping pills.

Tranquillising women

One fact has received very little attention from either the media or the medical profession: twice as many women as men take tranquillisers, and twice as many women as men are hooked on them. We find this the most disturbing fact of all.

Many of the doctors we spoke to were aware that they prescribed these drugs to women more often than to men. We asked them which people take tranquillisers most often:

- The picture that pops into my mind is a young-to-middle-aged woman in a crisis, but it may be different for other doctors.

- Late twenties or thirties, that is when they seem to start. Females mainly. There is a whole group of patients who, even if you solve their problems, will only produce more. We do find that we get a patient who has a problem with her husband or son or daughter and we try to sort that out, then there is a housing problem and they don't pay the rent and they just go on from problem to problem and crisis to crisis.

- Women and the elderly mostly.

- More the groups of people who need support and who are not capable of overcoming their problems and who come to me for help. More women than men I'd think. There are a great many people with similar problems who would never come to me and would get over it themselves.

The scores of medical and psychological studies which we researched for this book often differed in their findings about many aspects of taking tranquillisers; but whether the study was carried out in Australia, Belgium, Canada, Britain, the United States, Sweden, Switzerland, Italy, Spain, Japan, the Netherlands, Germany, New Zealand, France or Denmark, the sex ratio held true: the number of women taking tranquillisers was always at least double the number of men.[4]

The figures for antidepressants are less consistent but the trend they indicate is very similar – two-thirds of people taking them are women.[5] One study[6] in Canada found that, among people between the ages of 20 and 30 taking antidepressants, women outnumbered men by eight to one.

Why? Why should more than 20 per cent of Western women have their problems bottled up in the form of a prescription for a tranquilliser, a sleeping pill or an antidepressant? Are women really so much more depressed, anxious and sleepless than men? Even if they are, do tablets really help them? How can women cope with these problems without taking pills?

Our attempt to find some answers to these questions resulted in this book. We drew a lot on our own experience and research with people taking tranquillisers and antidepressants: in our work we examine the short- and long-term effects of these drugs and how to help people to stop taking tranquillisers.

We also drew on the current scientific literature, which is often a minefield of debate and controversy, and we interviewed scores of people concerned – women who take pills or who had recently stopped taking them, doctors who prescribe them, professionals who try to help people without using drugs, and representatives from a multinational drug company which manufactures tranquillisers and sleeping pills.

The reasons for disproportionate use of prescribed drugs by women go far beyond the surgery and the problem is not solely the responsibility of doctors. In many cases, women turn to their doctors for help with problems that medicine alone cannot solve, but few doctors like to turn their patients away empty-handed. While many GPs have recently cut down the number of prescriptions they give for tranquillisers and sleeping pills, they often feel they have no real alternative to drugs when faced with patients who are emotionally distressed.

In this book, we are not advocating that pills should never be used. We feel that when someone is too severely anxious or depressed to be able to start coping with the actual causes of their distress, then drugs can be useful in breaking the vicious circle long enough for the patient to change her circumstances. But we do not believe that most women taking these drugs are in such extreme cycles of depression or anxiety. The vast majority do not have mental 'illness' which can be 'cured' by drugs and, for them, taking pills can create more problems than they had to start with.

In focusing on women, we do not intend to underestimate

the problems of men who are bottling it up. We feel that the information given and the issues raised in this book concern both sexes, especially as we are now witnessing a startling increase in drug use by one group of men in particular – the unemployed. Women, however, have for several decades formed the majority of those bottling it up.

A brief history

Women formed the majority of those defined 'mentally ill' long before drugs were available to treat such illness. A century ago, women's 'ravings' were often ascribed to 'diseases' of their reproductive organs. Psychological problems and personality disorders were often treated by removal of the ovaries. Hysteria was thought to be an exclusively female complaint caused by a 'disease' of the womb (*hystera* is Greek for uterus), and treated by ice packs and pressure on the ovaries.[7] All this changed in the early part of the century with Freud, whose thinking removed the key to female psychology from their reproductive systems and put it in their minds: our problems, he suggested, were not caused by the womb but by our inner conflicts and repressions. The management of women's psychological distress was transferred from gynaecologists to psychiatrists, but nevertheless remained in medicine.

Today, one in six of all women in Britain will spend some time during their lives in hospital because of a nervous breakdown. More than 90 per cent of psychiatrists are men; more than 60 per cent of psychiatric patients are women. Yet most psychiatric 'diagnoses' nowadays are not made by psychiatrists but by general practitioners, and it is GPs who prescribe the bulk of the tranquillisers, sleeping pills and antidepressants consumed in Britain.

Problems of addiction to tranquillisers and sleeping pills also have a history. Before the discovery of Librium, Valium and the other benzodiazepine drugs currently prescribed, barbiturates were used as tranquillisers and sleeping pills and

16

they were found to be highly addictive. In January 1958, Dr Elijah Adams wrote an article in *Scientific American* regretting that barbiturates had been prescribed too easily, too often and for too long. Most of what he said would apply today to our present use of tranquillisers and sleeping pills – and so, we think, would his conclusion:

> Biologists look forward to the day when progress in medicine will make all present drugs, including the barbiturates, obsolete. Better understanding and treatment of the personal and social causes of anxiety should reduce our present reliance on chemical aids to tranquillity and sleep. (p. 64.)

Instead of better understanding of the personal and social causes of anxiety, we were given new, improved chemical aids to tranquillity and sleep. Dozens of new benzodiazepine tranquillisers flooded the market as the drug companies competed for profits. There was little difference between most of these drugs. The cost to the British National Health Service (NHS) was staggering, and in April 1985 the British Government introduced a restricted list which allowed only seven benzodiazepines to be available on NHS prescription.

It had taken 20 years to realise that the new benzodiazepine tranquillisers were also addictive. History has repeated itself and may do so again as the drug companies are already searching for and testing new tranquillisers and sleeping pills which they hope will be less addictive than the benzodiazepines.

We have written this book in three sections. In the first part we explore the reasons why so many women are bottling it up. Part 2 gives detailed information about the drugs themselves, about their side-effects, and about what happens when you stop taking them. The third part gives advice on the alternatives to drugs and a detailed self-help programme for anyone who wants to come off tranquillisers.

Wherever possible, we have tried to give the views of both

women and doctors in their own words. All the accounts that follow are true but we have given all the people we interviewed fictitious names to protect their privacy.

Part I   Tranquillising women

2 Seven women's stories

Sally's story

My doorbell rang and as my eldest daughter opened the door my three-year-old little girl darted out under her arms. Within a split second, she was run over by a car. They told me I would have to wait for weeks and weeks to get these brain scans to know if she was going to be normal.

Before that happened I was quite easygoing: I wasn't a neurotic mum or over-protective. But when I got my little girl home from the hospital after two months, it hit me. I was feeling guilty. If the door bell rang, oh my God! I couldn't sleep well and when I did sleep I'd jump up hearing a car screech. So I went to my doctor and told him I was getting into a state with the children. He gave me Valium [a tranquilliser].

I took them for a month and when I'd finished them I got these symptoms. I felt a bit dizzy and a bit numb. When I was going to get the children from school I felt as though I was lifting up from the pavement and coming back down.

So I went back to the doctor and he gave me some different pills – Ativan [another tranquilliser]. I was on those for about five years and it just got progressively worse. I was dreamy, I started to feel very inferior and then I became very frightened of going out. I would have to take a pill in order to be calm and sit and have a conversation with somebody. I became very quiet and didn't have any interest in anything. I'm not kidding you. I was like a zombie.

I felt as if something else had taken over my brain. I used to feel as if there were creepy-crawlies running inside my head. I thought, maybe I'm going crazy – there must be something in the family going back years.

I kept all that a secret – especially the fear of going out – because I reckoned my husband was going to think I'm nuts. But he said to me, 'You've become a different person, Sally. You used to be full of beans, always happy, and you've become like a vegetable.' In the end he got so fed up with it all because his idea of things was just to throw all those pills in the dustbin and get on with it.

Sometimes I got cheesed off and said, 'Right. I'm not taking all those silly pills.' But in the end I had to take them because of the hallucinations and because I couldn't see straight. And I was so confused. I knew I was an addict but at the same time I thought I needed them.

Once I asked to see a psychiatrist. He sent me for a brain scan. He told me I had a nervous disease and gave me antidepressants to take with the Ativan. In the end I told my doctor that I wanted to stop taking the pills. Okay, I had a problem five years ago with my little girl but that's all gone now and the pills are making me worse. He didn't agree but said, 'Fair enough,' and reduced my dose of Ativan.

Over 12 months Sally gradually cut down her pills and went through a long and difficult withdrawal period. When she told us her story, she had not taken tranquillisers for a year and vowed she would never again take mood-altering drugs. She felt very bitter about having been addicted to prescribed drugs.

I was asleep for five years. But I feel great now and I think you should tell people reading your book how fantastic life is when you're off the pills.

Charlotte's story

Charlotte is a 31-year-old legal secretary who has two children. Just after the birth of her daughter six years ago, she felt depressed and was afraid to go out of the house.

The doctor said that a lot of women get it and it is because you have just had a baby. He said it could be a hormone imbalance.

He also said that I was a very neurotic woman. But I had never been neurotic before. Anyway, he gave me hormone tablets and the Ativan pills [tranquillisers].

I found the Ativan helped me tremendously at first. I suddenly felt like I wanted to go out. And gradually I pulled myself together. After quite a long time, about three years, on the Ativan, I thought I'm not like that any more. I don't need them. That was when I found I couldn't come off them.

Over the next three years Charlotte managed to cut down her dose of Ativan from three a day to just half a tablet a day.

I found I could not get off that last half. When I tried not to take it, I felt terrible – very on edge and shaky. I think a lot of it was psychological: just the thought that I had not taken even that half tablet. But I could not stand how I felt, so after a day or so I'd have to take a half again.

Then six months ago, everything got on top of me. My divorce came through. I think I realised then that I was totally on my own, bringing up two children. I felt as if I could not cope, everything sort of crowded in. My mother was quite ill at the time, and we had a big court case coming up at work. Instead of just taking it all as it came, which I usually can do, I felt very low, very depressed, tearful.

I increased to three Ativan tablets a day, but I still felt uncomfortable and slightly panicky when I went out. They were not helping at all. I was also put on Prothiaden [an antidepressant].

I do not like taking Ativan. It gets to the point where people say to me 'What do you want to drink?' and I say 'Orange juice' and they ask 'Why don't you drink?' and I can't tell them. When you know you're addicted to pills, it's just not on. I don't believe that I'm weak. I don't like to be beaten on anything. Looking back, I think that if the doctor had explained to me what was happening to me after my little girl was born I could have coped with it. I could have learnt to live with it without pills.

Charlotte still takes antidepressants but now with the help of a psychologist she is trying to come off tranquillisers.

Jane's story

Jane was depressed in her first year as a student at Cambridge University. Her doctor prescribed diazepam (Valium):

> The pills were the only way I got through student life. I've been on them even since but only when I need them. I take them whenever I'm depressed or when I think I'm going to get depressed in some situation, or when I feel tense. I never take them to sleep, I sleep like a log.
>
> Once I asked my doctor if I could see an analyst, but he said I couldn't get that sort of treatment on the NHS. In the end I went privately but I still kept on the pills. I never see the doctor now. I just ring up the surgery and get a repeat for diazepam along with my contraceptive pills every three months. I never go out without the pills – I have to have them there in my bag with my Alka Seltzers.
>
> They're very social things, these pills, you know. I'm always giving them to friends or people at work when they are depressed. They are wonderful then. Someone comes up to you all freaked out and it looks like I'm going to be stuck listening to all their hassles and problems for ages. But then I give them a diazepam and 15 minutes later they're off all smiles and tranquillity. They save hours.

Jane has taken tranquillisers for seven years now. She is a successful assistant producer for a television company.

Anne's story

Anne is 30 years old and has three children. After the birth of her last child four years ago, her husband left her.

> I was so down, so depressed. The doctor said I had post-natal depression and gave me Librium [a tranquilliser]. I took them for two years but I got more depressed. Then I read an advert in a medical magazine which said that Valium gives you peace of mind. So I went to a new doctor and got some Valium.
>
> The pills helped at first – they took all that emotional stuff out of me. I felt lousy in the morning until I took a pill. After I took a

24

pill, I'd wonder what I was panicking for. They made me feel relaxed. I could talk to the kids again. That's how I am. I just kept on taking them – repeat prescription after repeat prescription. I couldn't cope without them.

But the more I took, they didn't seem to work any more. I went up and up till I was on six a day, even though it was meant to be only three. I got depressed on them. I was getting worse and worse – I just felt like a walking tablet.

I wouldn't have anything to do with my family. I wouldn't talk to people; I wouldn't even take the kids to school in case I met someone. I used to go and hide in a corner away from everything. The children were going out of their minds too because they wanted to go to school.

Then they sent me a new social worker. She was nice, she cared, you know. She didn't like me just getting pills and never seeing a doctor, so she got a doctor to refer me to the hospital for therapy.

Anne went once a week to the hospital where she learnt relaxation techniques, crafts and typing. Other patients as well as psychiatrists and psychologists talked to Anne about her problems and gradually her Valium was reduced. In March 1983 she had been off Valium for two months and her injections were stopped.

It was a whole complete personality change. I felt like a woman again and not a thing. I had so much confidence in myself. My complexion changed, I looked my age again, instead of 40. I was mixing with neighbours, family, I was going out. I was playing with the kids.

In November 1983 Anne went to see her doctor to see if he could help her be rehoused from her fourth-floor council flat. He said he'd try, and gave her Lexotan (a tranquilliser) to keep her going in the meantime.

He didn't tell me it was a tranquilliser – he said he took it himself. Now look at me. I can't go through all that again.

Brenda's story

I was 26 years old at the time and my husband was in prison. Someone suggested I go shoplifting with them. It seemed a good idea because we were very short of money and I had three boys to bring up. Of course it wasn't a good idea and never is. When I got a three-month prison sentence they put me in a cell and, as they closed the door, I got acute claustrophobia. The walls were coming in, the window looked 10 miles away. I have never been so terrified in my whole life. I remember thinking that I could hear someone screaming and about 20 minutes later I realised it was me. That was the start of the Valium.

Brenda has taken tranquillisers and anti-depressants ever since and is now 43 years old.

I was aware that I shouldn't be living my life on pills, and I didn't like the fact that I was addicted.

Over the years she has battled with the claustrophobia and can now get into a lift and travel on the London Underground.

Last year I saw a TV programme which influenced me greatly. I decided to stop the Valium dead. It was awful. It's hard to describe: panic of unbelievable strength – you feel you want to run but where are you going to run to; you try to combat the panic, but you can't and find yourself popping a pill.

Gradually, under the advice of her doctor, she cut down her dose of Valium to 5mg a day.

If I get upset, if my husband is getting drunk on a binge for the whole day and I know he will come in all soppy and drunk I get very pent up and take another tablet. Understanding from other people helps because that makes you emotionally happy and you don't need so many tablets. If you get love and affection it conquers an awful lot.

I think Valium is a curse. But you can't take them off the market now because people like me are dependent on them.

Emily's story

I had a lot of tension with my husband. He used to drink and go out with his friends. He didn't want me with him. I was just like a bit of furniture. The only time he realised I was around was when he wanted sex and that really turned me off. He used to threaten me. I find sex revolting now. Then he was going out with another woman at the time I found my dad dead. It really was the last straw.

Emily, who was 45 when that happened, was prescribed a tranquilliser and an antidepressant. She has taken them ever since and is now 62 years old. Divorced some years ago, she lives in a two-bedroom council flat with her 40- and 32-year-old sons.

The boys have a bedroom each and I sleep on the settee in the front room [she sometimes takes extra pills when she is upset about something] because I don't want to get on top of the boys. Sometimes I go out to bingo and take it out on the caller.

The pills definitely help me because if I leave off them I am worse. I feel upside down.

Emily told us that she does not talk about her feelings or problems with anyone except her doctor.

You can't really talk to boys. They don't understand. My boys just say, there's always something wrong with you, Mum.

Kathy's story

I moved to London because I married a Londoner. Before that I'd been looking after my five younger brothers and sisters, which I liked doing. When I moved to London there was just me and my husband. I was 19 then and felt very lonely and very homesick.

I was put on blue pills first – the heart-shaped ones – and they gave me energy. I took those for about five years until I was pregnant. I was really happy having my daughter and didn't need any pills, but when she went to school I was on my own again and I felt

27

depressed. The first thing you do is run to the doctor and say 'I'm feeling down'.

That is when I went on Valium. I used to take 2mg tablets and then I had a bad turn of depression and got the 5mg ones and then I had the 10mg ones: three of those a day. Taking the tablets became a pattern of life. You get up in the morning and don't have the confidence to go out until you have taken your pill; then about dinner-time I would feel a bit tired so I'd have a pill. After that I'd be all right for the afternoon and then at night I'd have jobs to do at home so I took another one. They were wonder drugs. They seemed to cope with all my problems. I was on them for 15 years. In the end I realised I wasn't living: I was just existing. I felt as if I was drugged all the time. Then I started to knock them off and, over about three years, I cut down to half a tablet twice a day.

My old doctor died and the new one doesn't like giving pills. I was just beginning the change of life when that happened so I really needed something. But he only gave me 20 tablets. I made them last for three or four months, cutting them in half and then into a quarter. Finally I realised that what I was taking couldn't possibly have any effect so I stopped altogether. I felt very ill, very shaky and panicky when I was cutting down.

Since I have been off I feel much better and have real confidence. I feel like I used to feel before I was married. When I was on the tablets I just went on from day to day and didn't notice things around me. Now I notice the birds, plants, all these things just like when I used to live in the country. I feel alive again. I just feel I wasted all those years of my life on tablets.

3 Medicines for the mind

There's a huge poster down the road from where we work which lists tuberculosis, cholera, typhoid, TB and polio... Each disease has a thick red line through it, crossing it off because it is solved, because medical science has made it a thing of the past. At the bottom of the list is cancer and the one word: when? The message is clear: given enough time and money, medicines will cure every ill, even cancer.

Enormous breakthroughs in medicine throughout this century have led us to expect a future where all pain can be relieved and all diseases cured. But can this include the 'pains' of living, the ups and downs, the anxieties and the depressions of everyday life? Can these be seen as 'illnesses'? Are they 'diseases' of the mind which, like diseases of the body, can be cured by drugs? Shall we eventually see a poster crossing off anxiety, depression, insomnia and ending with unhappiness: when?

Sixty years ago, the idea of millions of people taking tablets for psychological problems might have made a good science fiction story. Today – at this very moment – as over 100 million people have a tranquilliser in their bloodstream, and several million swallow their daily antidepressants,[1] it has become a medical reality.

Over a million Americans and a quarter of a million British are addicted to tranquillisers and sleeping pills. Realising this, many doctors have recently stopped showering prescriptions for them on their patients like confetti. At the same time, however, most doctors feel that they have no real alternative to tranquillisers when faced with patients' emotional problems.

What are tranquillisers, sleeping pills and antidepressants?

Tranquillisers are pills which calm people down. Nearly all of them belong to the family of drugs called benzodiazepines; so do nearly all sleeping pills. Indeed, the main difference between tranquillisers and sleeping pills is that one is taken in the daytime and the other is taken at night.

Although they are all the same type of drug, tranquillisers and sleeping pills have many different 'trade' names given by the different drug companies which make them. The famous Valium has the most aliases. It's exactly the same drug as diazepam, Evacalm, Solis, Atensine, Valrelease, Diazemuls, and Tensium. And Mogadon has its *Doppelgängers* in the form of nitrazepam, Nitrados, Somnite, Surem, Remnos and Unisomnia. The enormous number of names for these drugs makes it very difficult to know what exactly is written on a prescription, so we have included a checklist at the end of this book. Throughout this book, we have used chemical (generic) names and where trade names are used, they are mostly British. A full list of American, Australian and British trade names is given on pp. 157–60.

Tranquillisers like Valium have only been around for about 20 years. The very first benzodiazepine, Librium, was introduced in 1961. Before that, barbiturates were given for anxiety and sleep problems. Although barbiturates are still used occasionally for these problems, they were found to be lethal in overdose and to be highly addictive. Despite the problems we now know of benzodiazepines, they ousted the barbiturates because they were seen as much safer drugs.

Antidepressants are completely different drugs. They are supposed to do what their name implies – act against depression. There are several types of antidepressant: the most common (called tricyclics) include amitriptyline (Domical,

Elavil, Lentizol, Saroten and Tryptizol) and imipramine (Tofranil, Praminil). These drugs are dangerous if an overdose is taken.

Another type of antidepressant (monoamine-oxidase inhibitors – MAOIs) includes Nardil, Parnate and Marplan. These are prescribed much less often than tricyclics because they can interact dangerously with other drugs and even certain foods. For example, while taking these pills, patients must not eat cheese, pickled herrings, broad bean pods, Bovril, Oxo or Marmite or drink Chianti wine.

Why are they prescribed?

Tranquillisers are medically accepted treatment for severe anxiety, for severe sleeping problems, for relaxing muscles, for epilepsy, for helping alcoholics withdraw from alcohol, and as sedatives before operations. In practice, they are also prescribed for many other reasons.

Antidepressants are the medically approved treatment for depression, unless it is so severe that electroconvulsive shock may be advised. They are also recognised treatment for children over six who wet their beds at night.

Tranquillisers are sometimes prescribed for physical rather than psychological problems. Drugs like diazepam (Valium) relax muscles and may help rheumatism or hypertension. Whether they are effective in treating physical complaints is still being debated by the medical profession.

The effects of stress on physical health have received publicity in the last few years, and we all know the stereotype of the workaholic who may well end with an ulcer or heart problem. Some people visiting their doctor and complaining of severe headaches, stomach problems, or pains in different parts of the body may be diagnosed as having a 'psychosomatic' illness. This doesn't mean that the patient is cheating or making things up. It means that a physical symptom has been caused by a patient's underlying anxiety, depression or tension.

- I had dreadful, thumping headaches. I went to the doctor and he wanted to know if I had any worries or recent upsets. I told him that my mother had died recently. He said it was probably stress and that I should have a course of Librium [a tranquilliser].
- I was having difficulty over a virus. It was going on for about five or six weeks. Eventually the doctor put me on Valium.
- I had tension in the back of my head and tightness in my chest. I'd never had it before. My husband was out of work and we had money problems. I was prescribed Inderal [a beta-blocker to treat the physical symptoms of anxiety] and Ativan [a tranquilliser].

It is fairly common for these drugs to be given to patients for certain physical and psychosomatic problems. One study in Britain[2] looked at a large group of people who had just been prescribed tranquillisers and anti-depressants. 40 per cent of the men and 30 per cent of the women had complained to the doctors of physical, not emotional, symptoms.

Diagnosis: anxiety or depression?

- Sometimes it is difficult to tell depression from anxiety. When I was at medical school we were taught about people in psychiatric hospitals with severe depression, and not about those with a mixture of depression and anxiety who come along to the surgery.
- The difference between anxiety and depression is not always clear. For the past ten years I have attended a course for general practitioners at my local psychiatric hospital to help me understand better my patients' emotional problems. Despite that, I am still fooled by patients who underplay their symptoms, and I do not always realise when I am dealing with true depression and not an anxiety state.

It is not surprising that many doctors are unsure when to prescribe tranquillisers and when to prescribe antidepressants. Often people have symptoms of both anxiety and depression. For example, when we are depressed we usually have problems sleeping, and when we are anxious we often feel depressed about not coping better with life. Most psychologists agree that there is so much overlap between anxiety and depression that it is meaningless to think of them as separate problems.

For doctors, however, it becomes important to try to distinguish between anxiety and depression because they see them as two different 'illnesses' which should be treated by two different kinds of drugs.

● The effectiveness of drugs for anxiety and depression depends on the doctor's ability to make a correct diagnosis, and on how deeply ill the patient is. It is the first diagnosis which is so important.

Some of the doctors we interviewed felt that there were clear differences between anxiety and depression, but most said it was often hard to distinguish the two.

● You rarely get anxiety without depression. You usually see a bit of both. Sometimes anxiety predominates and sometimes depression.
● Anxiety and depression are often mixed up. Often you find a mixture of the two.

One doctor said he depended on his patients for guidance: 'I ask them whether they think they are more anxious than depressed, or vice versa.

Faced with this overlap between anxiety and depression, doctors can try to decide which of the two predominates and prescribe for that. Alternatively, a tranquilliser *and* an antidepressant may be given to patients who are thought to be both anxious and depressed. Drug companies have recently identified a market here and are trying to develop combined pills which are meant to have both antidepressant and tranquillising properties.

When do moods stop and 'illnesses' begin?

We all feel anxious or depressed at times as problems in our daily lives make us tense or get us down. For most of us, these are moods we know will pass as we solve our problems or adapt to new circumstances. But when do anxiety and depression change from being moods, which we all experience, to being 'illnesses' that doctors treat with drugs? It is unclear just how anxious or how depressed someone has to be before a prescription is written.

How do doctors decide if a patient is distressed enough to need pills? The *British National Formulary* – a drug compendium produced six-monthly by the British Medical Association and the Pharmaceutical Society of Great Britain – gives this advice about tranquillisers:

> Although there is a tendency to prescribe these drugs to almost anyone with stress-related symptoms, unhappiness, or minor physical disease, their use in many situations is unjustified. They should be limited to patients whose anxiety is clearly handicapping, as when it interferes with their work, leisure, or family relationships. In children anxiolytic [anti-anxiety] treatment should be used only to relieve acute anxiety (and related insomnia) caused by fear (1984 (No. 8), page 134).

Since tranquillisers were first introduced, the range of 'problems' they are advertised as helping has increased so much that sometimes it seems that the prescription is written first and the problem is diagnosed afterwards. As one research doctor put it, 'The medical diagnosis is turned on its head and the reasoning becomes "You're a case of Valium, you'd better have some anxiety".'

Trauma tablets

For most people, anxiety and depression are not things they expect to live with all their lives. More often, people become anxious or depressed because of specific problems or bad experiences for which doctors have no pre-packed solutions:

- I feel that when the doctor writes *me* a prescription for Valium, it's to put *him* out of *my* misery.
- The day after my husband died, the doctor came to see me and brought me the Ativan [a tranquilliser] to help me sleep.
- My husband had another woman and she had his baby. He left me and that's when I went on Ativan, I took three a day.
- The doctor said I had had a very difficult time because when my first husband died I had all seven children to bring up on my own. He gave me sleeping pills.
- Yes, the mugging. I still have not got over it. That was in January 1981. He beat me up. I wasn't hurt that much, just bruised here and there. But I think it was more the shock. She put me on a lot of pills. I still won't go out unless I am with company.
- My husband was battering me and sexually assaulting me in front of the children. I told my doctor exactly what was happening and he told me to take Valium.

Clearly, a tranquilliser will not bring back a dead husband, make men more faithful to their wives, help bring up seven children, stop muggings in the streets, or prevent a man from battering and abusing a woman. In giving tablets to women in such situations, the most a doctor can hope for is to suppress their symptoms of distress. What else can the doctor do?

Tranquillising women: a feminist issue

Why are so many women bottling it up with tranquillisers and antidepressants? Are more women than men anxious, sleepless or depressed? Or do women cope with these problems differently from men? For example, some people argue that women go to doctors with emotional problems whereas men tend to drink more alcohol. Are men just less emotional than women, as classic stereotypes would have it? Or do men have less problems than women? Is it a genetic difference between the sexes? Is it something to do with a woman's life cycle –

menstruation, reproduction and the menopause? Does the fact that women live longer than men have anything to do with it? Do the sexes have different relationships with their doctors so that women are more likely to be seen as needing tranquillisers or antidepressants?

There are as many explanations of the sex difference in bottling it up as there are questions and there is more than one factor involved. Only by looking at the circumstances in which women find themselves turning to a bottle of pills can we begin to understand why so many of us run the risk of becoming dependent on drugs.

Although all sorts of women take tranquillisers and antidepressants, certain groups of women are prescribed these drugs more than other groups. The chances of being prescribed tranquillisers and antidepressants depend mainly on whether a woman is married, single, widowed or separated, on whether she has a paid job, on how old she is, and on how much support she gets from her family and friends.

Marriage: a risk to female tranquillity?

In Britain and the United States, being married greatly increases a woman's chance of being treated for a mental 'illness' – mostly depression and anxiety.[3] For men, the position is reversed: being married actually reduces their chances of being diagnosed mentally ill. Single men are more likely to be treated for depression and anxiety than married men; the opposite holds for single and married women.

Employment: a psychological bonus for women and men

It has always been accepted that 'a man needs a job'. The recent bout of large-scale unemployment in the Western world has led to the development of a whole 'psychology of the jobless' and, as a group, unemployed men are probably the highest consumers of tranquillisers and antidepressants.[4]

36

It is still not widely accepted that women need jobs for their well-being. There is still no 'psychology of the housewife' that explains why she is so susceptible to being labelled 'mentally ill'. Yet studies have shown that being without paid employment can be a risk to the mental health of women as well as men.

Having paid jobs outside the home seems to protect women from being diagnosed mentally ill.[5] This may seem surprising as we are often told of the stresses of running a job and a home – the harassed working mother who is torn between the pressures of paid work and running the house and family. On the contrary, however, it's the hassled housewife, with no role outside the home, who is more at risk of being diagnosed depressed, anxious or sleepless. Housewives consume more sleeping pills than women in any other job.

One study in Canada asked a cross-section of women whether they had taken tranquillisers or antidepressants in the previous two weeks and 11 per cent of women with full-time jobs, 19 per cent with part-time jobs and 25 per cent of housewives said yes.[6] Similar patterns are found throughout Britain and the United States.[7] The Canadian study found that besides paid work, having hobbies and interests which were based outside the home also reduced a woman's chances of being on drugs.

One national survey in America looked at the families of people who took tranquillisers and antidepressants.[8] They found that women living in traditional nuclear families were twice as likely as men to be taking these drugs. But in non-traditional families where, for example, the woman went out to work and the man stayed at home, the sex difference disappeared and men were just as likely as women to be taking tranquillisers and antidepressants.

A woman's age

Although at every age from 16 to 90 twice as many women as men are prescribed tranquillisers, older women are prescribed them more frequently than younger women.[9] This is partly because middle-aged and older women are often given tranquillisers as sleeping pills.[10]

Different people need different amounts of sleep: some feel fine on three or four hours a night, some need 11 or 12 hours, but most of us get by on something between those extremes. As we grow older, we often need less sleep. The magic eight hours, which we were brought up to believe will make us feel at our best, is a myth. Some people who are sleeping less as they age feel there must be something wrong, that if only they could get the full eight hours, life would be so much better and they would have much more energy to cope with tomorrow. Taking sleeping pills does not often have this effect. Often people feel 'hungover' rather than energetic after a night on a sleeping pill and, when taken regularly, the pills will stop working after a few nights unless a higher dose is taken, and that soon leads down the path to addiction.

Women live longer than men and so are likely to experience more losses in their lives. It may be the death of a loved one, children leaving home, the loss of our physical or mental abilities, even the loss of a part of our bodies through mastectomy or hysterectomy. Often, the crisis of a loss can lead women to ask for medical help, which usually comes in the form of tablets.

Pills for years

The longer anyone takes tranquillisers, the less their chances of stopping. That's true of men or women. We do not know yet whether taking antidepressants for a long time can 'hook' people on them in any way. It is probably true, however, that if someone feels the pills have 'cured' their depression they will be unlikely to cope with future depression without them.

In Britain, working-class and middle-class women are prescribed tranquillisers equally often but working-class women tend to take them for a longer time.[1] In Canada, drug use has not been found to relate to social and economic levels,[12] but little information is available as yet on exactly who takes the pills for years. One London study[13] looked at patients receiving a new prescription for antidepressants and/or tranquillisers. It recorded what happened to the patient over the following year. The more depressed or anxious the doctor thought the patient was at first, the longer they were given drugs. That was equally true of men and women. But women (and not men) going through difficulties (e.g. with their marriage, family or jobs, or a recent bereavement) also stayed on the drugs for exceptionally long periods.

Medicines for the mind

What are these 'illnesses' that we are fighting with tranquillisers, sleeping pills and antidepressants? What kind of 'disease' can it be that afflicts housewives more than women with paid jobs, that occurs twice as often in women as men?

Doctors are trained to think of emotional problems as if they were like physical problems – the doctor's job is to diagnose the underlying 'illness' from the patient's symptoms and to find the best way of curing it. So, just as a running nose and sneezing are symptoms of a cold, anxiety and depression are viewed as symptoms of an 'illness'. By treating emotional problems like physical illnesses, doctors imply that we are anxious or depressed because we have something physically wrong with us. The most popular suggestion is that certain chemicals in the brain and nervous system are either missing or not working properly. On that basis, it makes medical sense to prescribe a drug to attack the illness, correct the imbalances in the brain and therefore remove the anxiety or depression.

Physical changes in our bodies do occur when we are anxious or depressed. But they may be a *result* of the anxiety or depression, rather than a cause of it. There are cases where severe depression is known to stem from physical causes, but these are relatively rare. And just because pills can offer relief does not mean that emotional distress has a physical cause. After all, aspirin can cure a headache, but the head-ache may have been brought on by stress.

● I am divorced and bring up my son on my own. Recently my mother took ill and I had to spend all my spare time with her. I couldn't cope with everything I had to do, I was on edge all the time and I felt exhausted. It was as if the world was rushing past and I couldn't keep up. I was horrified when my doctor said I needed antidepressants. I have been through tough times but I have never taken pills. He said it is like having a broken leg and putting it in plaster until it heals.

Does this woman really have some underlying illness? Or is her problem just what she says it is – simply that she has too much to do with not enough time to do it and she feels on edge? Does she feel that way because there is something wrong with the chemicals in her brain? Or is it more to do with the troubles in her life?

The mind and the body are not separate, they affect each other's well-being and both are affected by the stresses and strains in our lives. Even if for the sake of argument we accept that stress and worry can eventually lead to chemical im-balances in the brain, the question still remains one of how best to tackle the problem – prescribing drugs to deal with imbalanced brains or finding ways of coping with the stress?

The medical model seems to put the proverbial cart before the horse. After all, can a chemical imbalance account for a condition that is made more likely by being unemployed?

We know that in most cases depression and anxiety are reactions to things that have happened in our lives or to fears about what may happen in the future. Drugs are not going to change our partners, jobs, children or housing; drugs cannot bring back the people we have lost. By prescribing drugs, the most a doctor can hope for is that the symptoms of anxiety or depression will be alleviated for a while.

In addition to the dangers of addiction to tranquillisers, which most doctors now recognise, and the fact that the drugs alone cannot cure the causes of depression or anxiety, there are other reasons why a doctor's attempt to help with drugs is usually a misplaced kindness.

When a doctor writes a prescription for tranquillisers, sleeping pills or antidepressants, it reassures the patient that her problem is now in the hands of a medical expert. Her distress is diagnosed as an 'illness' for which she is being given a cure – the problem is now out of her control. The message is that her depression or anxiety is not a normal reaction to her circumstances, but an 'illness'.

This can clearly affect how a woman perceives her own emotions, as Stephanie, who took tranquillisers from 12 years of age until the day before her 21st birthday, describes:

- I spent all those years seeing myself as a psychiatric case. Tranquillisers never relieved my depression but they did make me define myself as not normal, not like everyone else. I feel resentful now. As far as I'm concerned I was born again at 21.

One in five women in the Western world each year are diagnosed as psychiatrically anxious or depressed. Are all those women really 'not normal'? Is the imbalance in their minds or in their lives?

4 Women, anxiety and depression

So far we have been talking about the hundreds of thousands of women who go to a doctor for help with their psychological problems, but there are many more women – probably millions – who are living with depression and anxiety without ever asking for medical help.

To see why women are so vulnerable to these psychological problems, we have to go beyond the doctor's surgery. Researchers have shown that the majority of people who are coping with anxiety and depression are doing so without medicines. They also find that those who score highest on good mental 'health' are married men with jobs; those who score lowest are full-time housewives with children.

Women are between two and six times more at risk of depression than men; more married women than married men are anxious; two-thirds of agoraphobics are women. Why?

In one study,[1] a psychiatrist was asked to assess the mental state of 458 ordinary women living in London. Fifteen per cent of them were so severely depressed that the psychiatrist would not have been surprised to see them as outpatients of a psychiatric hospital and a further 18 per cent were considered to be borderline depressive cases. So, in all, that meant one in every three of those 'ordinary' women were measurably depressed. Yet, as a recent book on women and depression points out, nowhere is there mention of this 'epidemic' which is sweeping the Western world.[2] Is it because it is considered 'ordinary' or 'normal' for women to be depressed? Certainly, sexual stereotypes have implanted notions that women are

42

emotionally and psychologically frail. Men are portrayed as the strong and steady sex: unemotional, rational, unerring as they plod in a straight line through life's realities. Women are equally exaggerated as opposites of that caricature: unpredictable, prone to emotional outbursts, irrational, up and down and upside down as they take life's problems to their hearts instead of to their heads. And of course, there's always the question of our hormones. We are expected to be on edge or depressed at different times of the menstrual month and during the 'change', and to have the 'blues' after giving birth.

The weaker sex?

Whether it is because of our hormones or our brains, the picture that's painted is one of women as psychologically 'weaker' than men, which makes it natural that we should have more psychological problems than the 'stronger' sex. But women are not weak. Indeed, part of the reason why little attention is given to the vast numbers of depressed and anxious women is that most of them do not even stop work when mentally 'ill'; the meals are still cooked, the shirts ironed and the children cared for. These supposedly 'weak' women are still supporting the day-to-day needs of their families, sometimes at the same time as holding down a paid job outside the home.

If we look at what the 'weaker' sex actually does and is expected to do in relation to the facts of mental illness, a different picture emerges: facts like the increased chance of depression for women who are full-time housewives, or the higher risk of anxiety for married women, or the enormous rate of depression and anxiety among mothers of pre-school children. The alleged weakness of women is not inherent in the female sex but more a result of the different roles and identities we have to maintain as the supporting cast in a society engineered for the needs of men.

In the next few sections, we shall explain why women in certain roles are vulnerable to depression and anxiety. Being vulnerable does not mean we necessarily become depressed or anxious. Clearly, many housewives and mothers do not have these problems. Being vulnerable means that we shall probably be depressed if something bad happens in our lives and we do not have enough support from the people around us to help us through.

Housework: a mental health risk

Boring repetitive work that is never finished, seldom praised and often unnoticed unless it is not done; social isolation; no status; no union; no pay: the job description of a housewife. It is depressing even to think about. It has all been said before but it little alters the housewife's lot. Women may have made a little progress in recent years towards a more equal position in the labour market, but sexual apartheid still rules in most kitchens.

Research confirms what many women know – full-time housewives are more dissatisfied with life and more prone to severe depression than other women.[3] For working-class or low-income groups, the rates of housewife depression are especially high.[4]

- Some days I feel like I am in solitary confinement and this place feels more like a cell than a house. It's the routine that gets me down, the washing, ironing, cooking, washing-up – it doesn't matter how much you do there's only more of the same to do tomorrow.

- Women like me and others round here, we're very cooped up in the flats. Men can always go out – out to work, out at night, out at weekends. But we're here with the babies and kids spending half the time cooking and cleaning and hardly ever going out except to collect kids or take them somewhere or go shopping. It's the housework that gets me down. You see the children growing up and changing and that's nice but the housework never changes.

Some researchers[5] in the United States compared working wives with full-time housewives. The full-time housewives felt more anxious, worried, lonely and worthless than the employed wives, and that was true regardless of education or income levels. Research in Britain has found the same pattern. Working-class women, whose jobs are often low paid with little status, are happier, more satisfied with life, and less vulnerable to depression than full-time housewives.[6] In Canada, one study found that full-time work more than halved the chances of a woman's being depressed.

It is not difficult to understand why paid employment benefits women's mental health. Unlike housework, a job gives us money and self-esteem, so we no longer define ourselves as 'just a housewife'. A job usually means getting out of the house and having different people to talk with. The advantages we derive from a job depend on the kind of work involved, and women are still unequal partners in the workplace, dominating the low-paid, unskilled jobs. Most nurses are women, most doctors, men; most secretaries and typists women, most office managers, men; the list is endless. Even in predominantly female occupations, such as primary school teaching, men still have far greater chances of promotion. Unions remain mostly male territories, and few actively campaign on women's issues.

Many women try to fit their paid work around their unpaid work as mothers and housewives. As part-timers, they often have little job security and are the first to be made redundant in hard times. As the general level of unemployment rises, part-time work becomes even more scarce, which directly discriminates against enormous numbers of women with families. Women who have stayed at home until their children left school also find they are unwelcome when they try to return to work, even if they have a good number of years of working life ahead of them.

The psychological advantages for women in employment are clear. Monica Briscoe[7] recently summarised the results of research on sex differences in mental 'health' by first rejecting the idea that 'women need men in the same way that men need jobs'. Rather, to safeguard against depression and anxiety, 'women need jobs in the same way that men need wives'.

45

Motherhood: 'the most important job in the world'

Between 30 per cent and 50 per cent of mothers with pre-school children have been found to suffer moderate or severe depression and anxiety.[8] The rates are very high among low-income groups, and much lower for middle-class mothers who can often afford to pay for labour-saving devices and for help with housework and children. The number of children we have, as well as how young they are, also affects our chances of being depressed. Having three or more children under 14 years of age at home is one factor making women more vulnerable to depression.[9] A survey[10] in the Midwest of the States found that women with pre-school children were the most likely women of all to be depressed and that going out to work did not make any difference to their mental health.

Having a job outside the home, however, can protect mothers against depression, after their children reach school age. There is still an argument that mothers of pre-school children are in a Catch-22 situation. If they go out to work, they often shoulder the guilt of not being 'proper' mothers, of being 'selfish' in not giving up those vital first few years to be with their children.

How happy women feel in going out to work will depend on knowing that their children are well looked after in their absence. Most families nowadays live away from relatives and their extended families and that in itself has created problems for women who cannot call on their own mothers for help and support with children. More often, child care has to be paid for so we have to earn enough to be able to pay someone else – inevitably another woman – to look after our children while we work. Unfortunately for both sexes, most men still play a peripheral role in child care. Having children is not meant to affect a man's job in any way and even paternity leave is rare.

We were all brought up to believe that motherhood is our 'natural' role in life and that women who did not have children were somehow unfulfilled and even abnormal. Relatives smiled happily when we were little girls practising for the future by playing with our little plastic babies that never cried and that always went to sleep when we wanted them to. The reality of motherhood is never as simple or as wholly romantic as we were led to expect.

For most women, motherhood has its ups and down: its moments of pure bliss and fulfilment, its moments of utter frustration, with just about every other human emotion experienced in between those extremes. As mothers, we know our caring and love are so important, so needed by our children, but at the same time our accomplishments are often neglected or undervalued by society as a whole.

When our children are very young, mothering can mean relentless 24-hour shifts and extreme physical tiredness. It is especially hard for women who are single parents and those who are cut off from the world in bleak, modern housing estates or tower blocks where there are little community life, poor transport facilities and few shops.

Many 'experts' on child care have stressed the importance of the mother–child relationship but are concerned with only one side of it – the child's. The mother's needs are largely ignored. In the textbooks she exists to cater for her infant's every need, producing breasts on demand, stimulating, comforting and entertaining her child from day one on. She is there to establish that crucial mother–child 'bond', that maternal super-gluing without which, we are told, all psychological hell will be let loose on the infant. Often, however, she is going through her own private mental hell and there are no textbook solutions for deprived mothers. As Ann Oakley[11] points out in *Subject Women*, there is no other job that combines such total responsibility, long hours, lack of pay and lack of social support to make victims of us women who, we are told, are doing the 'most important job in the world'.

Playing our 'natural' role in life, we are expected to adapt to being a mother without problems. Our mothers did it, our husbands' mothers did it, most women do it, so why should we complain? For some women, the birth of a first child brings an identity crisis, especially if they have recently stopped working. The first baby can mean a loss of freedom and control over the world, as a woman's needs and wishes now have to adapt to those of a child. Many women feel resentment at having to cope with all the demands of housework and a family and if those feelings have to be suppressed it is not surprising that many women feel helpless, hopeless and, in the end, depressed.

The problem is not solved when the children eventually grow up and leave home. After 20-odd years of caring for children, a woman who has been a full-time mother/housekeeper may feel empty and useless. If we are no longer needed we can feel a sense of worthlessness which may develop into depression.

Troubling times: depressing experiences in our lives

Many women we interviewed began taking tranquillisers and antidepressants after a traumatic event or distressing experience in their lives. In many cases this involved a loss of some kind.

Loss can take many forms – the death of a husband, child or parent is an obvious example. Society recognises how important it is to give sympathy and support to the bereaved. People expect a widow to feel depressed and to go through a long period of grieving before she can adjust to her new life. Friends and relatives will try to offer her comfort, help and understanding.

It is quite common for doctors to step in and give the recent widow 'something to help her sleep' or 'something to calm her nerves a little'. Although aiming to help, the doctor may be hindering the widow's adjustment in the long term. Not only may it place her on the slippery slope of tranquilliser addiction, but research[12] has also shown that it is necessary for a widow to go through the full emotional process of grieving for her loss. Tranquillisers may 'numb' her emotions and delay the inevitable grief.

There are many other forms of loss and separation besides death. Separation from loved ones, divorce, children leaving home, and unemployment, can all imply loss. There are physical losses when breasts or wombs are removed or when faculties are lost with age, disease or accident. Loss challenges our self-identity and our sense of being able to control our lives. Violence does the same – women who have been raped, physically abused or physically threatened have also lost in a very fundamental and painful way their own sense of power over events in their lives.

Unlike death, there are no rituals associated with these and many other forms of loss, nor is there a socially accepted period of grief. We are expected to cope, but if we do not have other people's support at such times in our lives, we may well end up severely depressed or anxious.

Emotional support

Research has shown how women who have little emotional support are more likely to have psychological problems.[13] The main safeguard we can have against becoming severely depressed or anxious is people we can turn to with our problems. Friends, husbands, lovers, workmates, relatives, neighbours, priests and doctors can provide a listening ear and sympathy in difficult times.

This kind of emotional support is something women are generally good at giving. As children, we learnt that women are meant to be caring and giving. It was mainly women who looked after us as children (mothers, babysitters, minders and most primary school teachers) and from them we learnt the feminine art of self-sacrifice – how to be sensitive to the needs of others, and how not to be selfish by doing only what we wanted to do. Similarly, in very subtle ways, we learnt that self-assertiveness and aggression were 'unfeminine'.

Nurtured in these days, women develop acutely sensitive

emotional antennae with which they can respond to other people's psychological needs. This is surely one reason why married men are such a mentally healthier group than single men. Wives are generally skilled at providing an often invisible emotional back-up service for husbands. But often there is no one in the nuclear family to respond to the needs of the mother and wife.

- Men go home and moan to their wives and then the wives end up at the doctor's surgery. The man is made redundant or has work pressures and the wife ends up on drugs. (Rose)

Like Rose, some women felt they were on drugs because of the pressure of other people's problems. Jennifer, however, told us how she had coped with her husband's anxieties in another way by prescribing *her* tranquillisers for *him*:

- My husband was tense because there were problems at the office. His job was on the line for months and he was hell to live with. I told the doctor I was all nerves and got the Valium. I never took one, ever. I just put a pill in my husband's cup of tea every morning. It worked a treat. He still doesn't know to this day.

Jennifer was prescribed Valium for two years and never told her doctor what she did with them. Passing the pills in this way may be quite common – several other women we spoke to explained how they sometimes gave tranquillisers to relatives or friends.

As wives and mothers, women are depended on by husbands and children for their emotional welfare. We nurture and support our families so that children grow up secure and happy. We adjust the emotional temperature in our homes so that husbands after a bad day at work don't get over-heated by the children climbing all over them or having the TV on too loud. We do all this usually without being asked and often without realising why we are doing it. Some women have husbands and children who do the same for them, but many do not.

Self-awareness

● I think it is very much the type of life women have – caring for others and having the responsibility of caring for others. They do the worrying about health whether it's their children or their husbands or themselves. There is a constant awareness of health by women. You see it reflected in women's magazines – they always have health articles – but men's magazines seldom do. Women are much more aware of their feelings and their bodies. (Dr B.)

Studies in Britain[14] and the United States[15] find that when people feel vaguely distressed – 'all on edge', 'ratty', 'not myself', 'fed up', 'a bit low' – women are much more likely than men to be aware of an underlying emotional problem, and to self-diagnose psychological problems. Men are less likely to analyse their own feelings, which may mean problems get worse in the long run. And men often vent their emotions in aggression at work or drown them at the pub. When home and workplace share the same address it is much more difficult for women to find similar emotional escape routes. This, together with women's increased self-diagnosis of emotional problems, is part of the reason why more women go to their doctors for help and return with a prescription.

So women's sensitivity is a double-edged sword. It is clearly an advantage to the people we support and care for, but, by diagnosing our own emotional problems, too often we are saying 'there's something the matter with *me*'. Often, however, we fail to recognise that the problem is not just in our heads, it's in our lives.

When the demands of housework, motherhood and often a paid job combine so that we feel everything is on top of us and we cannot cope, many women feel there is something wrong with them – they need a 'tonic' to pep them up or a Valium to calm them down. So, if the traditional female roles become hard to fulfil, then many women question their own mental health before questioning the roles they have to play. Even if we do recognise that our problems stem from our lives, many of us feel it does not help because we think we cannot change things anyhow. These feelings of helplessness only contribute to depression. Many women, having put the needs of others first for so long and their own needs always at the bottom of the list, no longer know how to say what they need.

There is no question that many thousands of women are prescribed pills for problems which are not medical or even simply personal, but social. And it is no coincidence that a large proportion of tablet takers are women who are bringing up children on an inadequate income in inadequate housing. By treating these women's reactions to their social situation as an 'illness', it is the women themselves who are seen as inadequate, and not their situation. Yet there is no doubt that social disadvantage increases the likelihood of anxiety and depression and even some government ministers might agree:

● Some activities, some social structures, and some family patterns seem to be helpful to mental health, in other words they reduce the likelihood of problems, and reverse ones are harmful. . . . We need to involve the whole of society with concerns about unemployment, about housing, about the environment, about education and so on, and also to make institutions that now exist – the Government included – far more sensitive to mental health issues. (*Minister for Health, 1981.*)

Since 1981 an increase in unemployment, an increase in poverty, and a decrease in our social services, have exacerbated emotional distress rather than relieved it, and many doctors feel that there is little they can do.

● I do not think that doctors can change the world.
● I get a bit annoyed when they want to involve me in housing because I really feel that I cannot do much about that. It is not my department.

But not all feel that way.

● I had a patient with twins who was living in a little flat and I got her a big house with a big garden. Since then she has settled down

52

very nicely, and it may just make the difference between popping into the surgery all the time and being able to cope.

● It is the continuous grind of having three kids in a flat that gets women down. I think that day nurseries and other kinds of help are alternatives to drugs.

Pills are certainly no answer in these circumstances, and their use for social problems has been described as 'a prescription for adjustment', because taking them will make us feel less like struggling to change the situation which upset us in the first place.

When faced with problems, whether they are caused by our social disadvantages as women or by personal trauma, where do we find comfort if it is not available in the home? Years ago we might have turned to near-by relatives or the church. Today it is more likely that we pay a visit to the doctor's surgery.

5   Women and doctors

What happens when we take our problems to our doctors? A lot depends on the individual doctor. They vary enormously in the numbers of tranquillisers and antidepressants they prescribe. There are also enormous differences in doctor–patient communication. Some feel that a prescription for these drugs is often an excuse for not listening to a patient's problems. Others feel that time pressures and lack of training in dealing with emotional distress mean they often have no real alternative to drugs.

In this chapter we shall look at the patient–doctor relationship from the viewpoints of both women and doctors.

Double standards?

● Most doctors are men, most patients are women. I have no doubt that there are some paternal, protective and sexual feelings between doctors and patients that make male doctors think they must help women more [than men]. I think that women are also under far more stress than men basically in a sexist society.

It's also something to do with the way men present themselves. It is a sort of macho thing; they are less involving, more matter-of-fact: here's the problem and let's see what we can do about it. I feel that prescribing for men is not as urgent or so necessary. Men talk about problems in a different way. I suppose the one benefit of a macho approach to things is that they tend to say 'I don't need tablets, I can manage it myself. (Dr M.)

This London GP was aware of how differently he responded

to men and women patients. For some physical problems, this is obviously necessary but it is not obvious why doctors also treat us differently for emotional problems.

When men and women report similar psychological or psychosomatic symptoms, men are more likely to be given physical tests and further treatments, whereas women are more likely to be given drugs. And once they have been prescribed antidepressants and tranquillisers, women are more likely than men to be given a series of repeat prescriptions.[1]

Doctors diagnose more women than men as anxious or depressed, and the reason is not simply that more women than men have emotional problems. In a study[2] of 91 GPs and over 4000 of their patients, the doctors were found to be more likely to diagnose anxiety and depression in women than in men, even among those who would not be considered to have an emotional problem according to a standard psychiatric rating. Young, educated, unmarried men who were anxious or depressed were particularly likely to be overlooked.

As one doctor we interviewed commented:

● Male patients do not involve your emotions in the same way, and I am sure there are also more complicated reasons, like not wanting to get close to someone of your own sex.

One reason for the differences in diagnosis between the sexes is that the 'symptoms' which doctors use to diagnose anxiety and depression are more common in women than in men. More women than men do not like going out, and because this is seen by doctors as a 'symptom' of an 'illness', more women than men are diagnosed as having this 'illness'.

Women and men as patients

As women, we need to consult our doctors far more often than men. Apart from the odd check-up or vaccination, men only visit a doctor when they are ill and probably needing a sickness certificate. Women, on the other hand, often go to their doctors when they are perfectly healthy. During our 30 years of fertility, we depend on doctors for the most basic control of our bodies. Doctors provide contraception, and sanction abortions; they check us for breast and cervical cancer; they monitor and care for our healthy bodies in pregnancy and childbirth. In our role as family health watchers, we have additional contact with doctors when we take our children or elderly relatives to the surgery. So doctors play a more regular and wide-ranging role in a woman's life than they play in a man's.

- Until recent times – because unemployment now plays an important part – men felt it was a sign of weakness to come to the doctor and confess they were sleeping badly or that they were irritable or that they were having domestic trouble. Men would not admit it. They are doing it more now, but women will come more readily. (Dr R.)

Many men feel a sense of failure in asking for help with psychological problems; they think they should be able to cope with such things themselves. Taking pills does not have a manly image either, especially when the pills are for the 'nerves' rather than a physical illness. Men use alcohol more than women, having a few drinks to calm them down or a night-cap to help them sleep.

- The men are the breadwinners and out at work they have avenues for getting rid of hang-ups and problems – partly by burying themselves in work, partly by going down to the pub for a pint. A lot of housewives don't have this opportunity – they can't get away from their problems. (Dr F.)

Women on doctors

- I get worried in case he thinks I'm not bad enough to go.
- I sit in the waiting room and rehearse what I'm going to say.
- He's always looking at his watch. He makes me feel that I'm wasting his time.

Many women are concerned that they may be wasting the doctor's valuable time when they go to the surgery. And many worry that the doctor will think they have come for a trivial reason. Because they are the 'experts' most of us feel unequal in our conversations with doctors. The doctor can call us Val or Sue but we can't call him Harold. We ask for help, the doctor 'gives'. Most doctors do most of the talking.[3] We tell them our symptoms, they decide what is and isn't relevant to the diagnosis. And for most of us, the doctor is from a different social and intellectual world:

● Sometimes we are thought heartless by the patients because there is a gap between our experience and theirs. But the doctor must try to close that gap and to find out what is really worrying the patient. (Dr D.)

This difference in knowledge separating patient and doctor is made greater by the secrecy surrounding our medical records. These are the history of every contact we have had with doctors from birth on, but we are not allowed to see them. These secret records can label patients as hypochondriacs (people who are always imagining illnesses), neurotics, anxious or depressed and, as these records are passed from doctor to doctor, it is difficult for us to lose those labels. So having once been prescribed tranquillisers, a woman going to her doctor complaining of severe headaches or backaches may well find her problems diagnosed as psychosomatic without any physical examination taking place. Often a doctor will not even tell her he thinks her problems are really psychological, so she is not given the opportunity to question.

Women are generally reluctant to criticise their doctors and tend to excuse and justify any faults they might find. In a study of the relationship between women and doctors, Helen Roberts[4] found that women who felt satisfied with their doctors praised their 'bed-side manner', saying they were nice to talk to, had time to listen and would come out to their homes in emergencies. Women who were not satisfied with their doctors nevertheless excused them by saying 'how busy' or 'how clever' they were.

Many of the women we interviewed felt that their doctors should have explained the risks of tranquilliser addiction and some felt the initial diagnosis had been wrong, yet they repeatedly excused these failings by emphasising how little time the doctor had or how reliable he was in other areas of medicine. As Marion explained, this is often because women do not want to antagonise their doctors, on whom they rely:

● My doctor is in his late forties and he has quite a good name in the area. Other things I went to him for he's fine. But on the question of tranquillisers, he still believes you can take them till you're 80 and they will do you no harm whatsoever. I never told him what I went through coming off [tranquillisers] or that I never had a nervous disease in the first place. I won't tell him because I still take the kids to see him from time to time.

Despite their experiences with tranquillisers and sleeping pills, few women shared the disillusionment of Joan, who had been taking Valium for 19 years:

● I had great faith in my doctor. I really thought she was terrific. Not any more. It's like you have no rights with doctors. You are the ignorant person, the layman, and you have no right to know anything about your own body.

The right to know?

On the basis of their medical knowledge, doctors make a diagnosis and decide on the treatment. How much the patient is told about that process – about how the diagnosis was reached, what the treatment entails or what problems there may be with the drugs prescribed – depends on the doctor. Most of the doctors we interviewed for this book felt that the dangers of addiction to tranquillisers and sleeping pills should be explained to patients, but discussing anything else depended on the individual patient.

- I always explain things to patients. That's part of what I call family practice.
- I think patients should be told as much as they want to know about medicines.
- I tell them the bad things about benzodiazepines.
- I give them a simple explanation, a little white lie sometimes.
- I usually tell patients that the pills are not the answer and that they will only trim the edges off an acute crisis. A lot of patients' problems are insoluble.

Not all doctors shared those views:

- Someone was saying people should be told all about the side-effects and dangers of the drugs. I think this is absolute nonsense. I wouldn't prescribe a drug if I didn't think it was necessary.
- There is no need to increase the patient's anxiety by telling them all sorts of weird and wonderful side-effects that they might experience and the fact that they might become dependent. It's counter-productive.

Counter-productive for whom? This kind of paternalism is quite common. An American survey[5] found that 54 per cent of doctors did not want their patients to receive information sheets or package inserts with their drugs, most of them claiming that patients would not understand and would be confused by them.

Patients often remember little of what went on in the surgery, especially if they felt anxious at the time. Doctors may think they had given explanations when they actually communicated very little to the patient, as one doctor had discovered:

- We have done some films of ourselves and patients and we are actually appalled at the way in which we have conveyed information to patients. It's virtually non-existent. We think we are doing it but how much the patient actually acquires is another matter.

Women doctors

Are women doctors more sympathetic to emotional problems?

Many of the women we spoke to felt the sex of the doctor made little difference, and some older women preferred men doctors because they thought they were more authoritative. A few thought that women doctors were less sympathetic than men because women doctors, like their women patients, had the problems of running a home and a job. Those who had been prescribed drugs during the menopause, after the birth of a child, or at the onset of menstruation felt that a woman doctor would have understood the problem better and been less likely to prescribe tranquillisers.

● I think male doctors believe that a lot of these things women go to them about are either imaginary or you are making them out to be worse than they really are. They've no idea what it's like because they are not women. I'm in an all-women practice now and the approach is completely different. They are more prepared to listen to you and more prepared to refer you if they feel the problem needs further investigation.

Men seem to prefer women doctors, too, for certain problems. A British study[6] of 4000 patients and 91 doctors found that when men had psychological problems they were more likely to choose to see a female doctor in a group practice.

Women doctors are still a minority in a profession where men are most definitely at the top. Sexual discrimination is most severe in hospital medicine and less in general practice where part-time work allows some women to spend time with their children as well as their patients. The lack of women in top medical jobs is even more striking when we realise that, on the whole, women out-perform men at medical school examinations.

Women have fought more keenly for places in medical school and it is well established that their performance in examinations has been better than men's. Unfortunately, women's academic performance while students is not proportional to their persistence as full-time medical practitioners.[7]

The excuse is always the same – women might have babies and that means less value for money than men. A profession which is dominated by men and which discriminates against its own female professionals is unlikely to treat its male and female patients as equals.

The doctor's view

● The problem has become so much greater in the years that I have been a doctor. Today the doctor is the person that the patient comes to first rather than ask friends, neighbours or the vicar or the social services.

A doctor's job has changed dramatically in the past 35 years that Dr Albert has been a GP. With the break-up of extended families and of close housing communities and with fewer people looking to religion for comfort and advice, doctors have found themselves taking on the roles of priest, neighbourly adviser and father figure as well as their traditional role as 'healers of the sick'.

Doctors did not ask for these extra roles, but few refuse to accept them. They do not like to turn patients away and say 'This is not a problem I can help with.' A doctor working in general practice needs a very wide range of skills and knowledge, for which he is trained only in part at medical school. A doctor's training in matters of emotional distress is particularly lacking.

● I don't think anyone mentioned emotional problems at all when I was a medical student.

● We did one year psychiatry, but psychology wasn't dealt with at all, sex wasn't dealt with at all and stress wasn't dealt with at all.

61

- We were trained by hospital doctors and the situations and the problems are completely different. Hospital psychiatry really has very little relevance to general practice where we are dealing with emotional distress rather than psychiatric problems.

This lack of education is not confined to Britain. A survey[8] in the United States reported that two-thirds of the doctors interviewed felt that their training in anxiety and depression had been sparse or non-existent throughout medical school, internships and residencies.

Many doctors believe that psychiatry is badly taught partly because it is never taken quite as seriously as other areas of medicine (psychiatrists are often known as 'trick-cyclists' in medical school). Without a proper training in dealing with emotional problems, and with only a short time to give each patient, it is not surprising that so many GPs find themselves reaching for the prescription pad.

- We are not trained very well in issues of this sort so it's easier to prescribe than counsel.

Explaining our emotional problems takes time, and a doctor may feel he has not enough time to listen. Writing a prescription for something is the traditional end to a visit to the doctor. On average, a British GP has only six and a half minutes to spend with each of his patients.[9] So it is easy to see why doctors with a queue in the waiting room may feel tempted to prescribe as a way of stopping a long and upsetting consultation. More than two-thirds of all visits to doctors result in a prescription.

- Each doctor makes his own play-off between the therapy he wants to give and the time he has available to give it.
- You cannot always blame the doctor. The fact is the doctor has not always got the time. Because of the pressure of the number of people in the waiting room, you may take the line of least resistance.

Some patients ask for a prescription and feel dissatisfied if they are refused.

● If you have a surgery of 30 people and someone comes in wanting sleeping pills you are not going to spend 15 minutes explaining why they should not have them. It's much easier to give them.

For the patient, a prescription is seen as 'proof' of her 'illness'. ('If I need pills, I must be ill.') It means she was right to go to the doctor, and had not wasted his time. Some doctors may try other ways of helping the patient but, if they do not work, a prescription can be a last resort:

● Say you reassure patients, explaining things to them and they keep coming back. After a time you feel defeated. The temptation is to say 'Take this'. Sometimes I find myself giving tranquillisers as a sort of admission of failure.

Such is the power of a prescription and the pills it brings that, in many cases, patients feel better simply because they *expect* to feel better. If those pills contain nothing more powerful than sugar, two in every five anxious or depressed patients will improve *as much as* when the pills are antidepressants or tranquillisers.[10] So for 40 per cent of patients, it's not the drug itself that makes them feel better so much as their *belief* that the pills will help.

What doctors learn after medical school: the lessons from drug companies

After a doctor qualifies, he still needs to keep up with new developments in drugs, diagnosis and other medical techniques. He can read medical journals, he can attend conferences and workshops, and he can join special-interest groups.

One main source of information for doctors is the drug companies themselves – mostly large, mostly multinational organisations which develop, test and sell drugs to the world.

Each of these companies sends representatives to visit doctors and there is one drug representative for every seven GPs in Britain.[11]

Drug companies also send free journals and promotional materials to doctors. On average, a GP is exposed to 300 drug company advertisements every week.[12]

Their lack of training in problems of anxiety, insomnia and depression makes doctors far more susceptible to the drug companies' information on those problems. Some drug companies claim that the education of doctors is one of their main functions. Drug companies are also in business, however, and their aim is to make profits by persuading doctors to write prescriptions for their particular brand of sleeping pill, tranquilliser or antidepressant. Many doctors therefore find themselves trained in emotional problems less by medical schools than by drug companies; and drug companies cannot make profits from doctors counselling their patients or teaching them relaxation techniques.

● Education is probably one of the best ways of promotion. You must remember that we are in business to make a profit so that we can plough that back into research and develop compounds for the future. (Marketing manager, multinational drug company.)

Drug companies also provide finance for the medical profession. Income from drug advertisements provides 43 per cent of the American Medical Association's total funding.[13] The drug industry supports medical lectureships, meetings, conferences, dinners, parties and all kinds of social events for doctors and medical students. Within universities and hospitals it funds drug trials which test and compare the effects of different drugs. All this means that the medical profession is partly dependent on drug companies for finance and sponsorship. The drug companies are clearly dependent on doctors who prescribe their products, and so the relationship between the pharmaceutical industry and medical professionals is mutually supportive.

Drug advertising

> As I look at the current advertisements for these drugs I cannot but feel some shame; partly I am disturbed that the pharmaceutical industry should use advertisements more suitable for cosmetics than for drugs, but mainly I am ashamed that such advertisements should be successful in influencing members of a learned profession. (GP researcher.)[14]

The information from drug companies ranges from their glossy advertisements, which would look at home in *Vogue* magazine, to sophisticated journals, tape-slide shows and videos. However educational and informative these may be, their aim is to persuade doctors to prescribe certain brands of drugs.

Advertisements often show pictures of the target patients for a particular drug. For example, promotional material for antibiotics will show a range of people, young and old, male and female, but in advertising for antidepressants and tranquillisers, pictures of women outnumber pictures of men by 15 to 1.[15]

It is hard to see how doctors could fail to be influenced by the barrage of advertisements they see and the stereotypes of patients pictured in them. For tranquillisers and antidepressants, there are enormous numbers of advertisements because of the huge competition between companies for the market in these drugs. Here are a few recent examples from some highly respected professional medical journals (*American Journal of Psychiatry, British Medical Journal* and *Australian and New Zealand Journal of Psychiatry*):

When depression disrupts the day

A middle-aged woman stands at a stove, a pan is boiling over and tears trickle down her cheeks. (Advertisement for Norpramin – an antidepressant.)

Life situations can take a turn for the worse

A divorce certificate from the Supreme Court of the State of New York is screwed up and over it is superimposed a picture of a beautiful young blue-eyed blonde woman looking sexy but sad. (Advertisement for Asendin – an antidepressant.)

Fast asleep all night, wide awake all day
A middle-aged woman holds two pictures of herself next to her face. In the picture on her left she looks anxious, on the right she looks half asleep. In the middle, she is smiling.
(Advertisement for Noctamid – a sleeping pill.)

Depression hurts
A young woman sits at a dressing table but can't bear to look in the mirror. (Advertisement for Merital, an antidepressant.)

Tears and fears
A middle-aged woman stares into space as tears cascade from her eyes. (Advertisement for Ativan, a tranquilliser.)

When depression disrupts the day
An attractive young typist is in floods of tears as she sits at her typewriter with audio-cassette headphones on.
(Advertisement for Norpramin, an antidepressant.)

Implicit in many such advertisements is the message that drugs can help women cope with their traditional roles in life: depressed because a pan is boiling over or depressed because she is not looking at herself in a mirror? Another advertisement shows a pretty young woman walking down stairs carrying a full laundry basket. The caption reads, 'In depression – first get the patient moving.' Yet another shows a young blonde woman collapsing into an armchair still wearing her nightdress: 'Some days she can't seem to function . . .', and promotes a tranquilliser.

We asked a drug company about this use of traditional female stereotypes in advertising:

- Yes, but they are the patients if you look at the patient population. How appropriate is [an advertisement showing] a young man with children? Obviously there are an increasing number of fathers who don't go out to work and who take over the maternal role but they are not something that the GP would simply identify with. (Marketing manager.)

Most advertisements occupy a whole glossy page in the journal. Information about the drug, which the drug companies are obliged to give with advertisements, is generally in very small print on another page. Some are more subtle, like the gleaming silver brain selling Xanax (a tranquilliser); or the picture of a beautifully calm woman with two little circles on her brain – one black, one gold – and you are not sure if they are meant to show the sun coming out of an eclipse or a golden pill beaming serenity on her brain (Desyrel, an anti-depressant).

Some advertisements show men, and these are often of the 'X will help you work, rest and play' genre, showing middle-aged executives who before 'X' look harassed by mountains of paperwork but after 'X' appear calm behind a cleared desk-top.

Elderly people feature a lot, especially in advertisements for sleeping pills. A smiling old lady clambering on to a bicycle is headed 'Restoril (a sleeping pill) gets along very well with most older patients'. The back cover of every issue of the *American Journal of Psychiatry* in 1984 showed a giant hand protectively cupped around a pipe-smoking gentleman looking out over some rolling hills. We are urged to 'Trust Tranxene' (a tranquilliser) and told 'Tranxene helps keep you in control of therapy'.

The way drugs are advertised varies from country to country, some using national events to promote their products. For example, we were given an advertisement at a conference which said in huge letters 'Normison made it with flying colours in the Falklands'. Normison was not a British officer in the Falklands' war: it is a sleeping pill.

Are drug companies indoctrinating doctors to prescribe their drugs? We asked a psychiatrist who is working in a multinational drug company:

● We advertise to promote our own products and as there are a lot of products, there is a lot of advertising. You could say that this is indoctrinating the GP to over-prescribe. I feel it is not. If you are exposed to a lot of toothpaste advertisements do you actually use more toothpaste than anyone else?

The analogy is an unhappy one as toothpaste is not, as far as we know, addictive nor is it available only by prescription or advertised exclusively for doctors.

● Most people when faced with advertisements look at them for perhaps two or three seconds. It is the same process as advertising consumer goods except that we are advertising, let us hope, in a more ethical and a more controlled way. But you are still trying to put your product in the appropriate niche for that doctor.
(Marketing manager, multinational drug company.)

Drug companies point out that they have to adhere to a Code of Practice when advertising their products, and that they are very strictly controlled in terms of what they can and cannot say. But there is no clear dividing line between deception and distortion. The advertising material which is presented to doctors may not be false, but it may mislead them to believe that the drug is something that it is not. Most doctors have a lot of personal experience of prescribing diazepam, so when a new tranquilliser is put on the market it is compared with Valium. But often doctors do not have the statistical knowledge to enable them to understand just how different the two drugs really are. They are dependent on the drug companies to tell them about the new product and, not surprisingly, drug companies are often rather selective in what they choose to say.

Images used in advertisements depict a drug as one answer for women who find their lives miserable, who cry at the cooker or who cannot face the housework. Dissatisfaction with our lot as housewife or secretary becomes translated into an illness which can be treated by drugs. The problems of living are very subtly advertised as coming under the umbrella of medicine.

Are pills the answer? The sexual politics of health

Few people would disagree that there has been a great deal of over-prescribing and mis-prescribing of pills for emotional problems, particularly for women. This has happened much more with tranquillisers than with antidepressants because tranquillisers were thought to have fewer side-effects and to be safer, and for that reason were welcomed as the answer to all our problems – both the doctor's and the patient's.

Recent articles and books by journalists about the effects of tranquillisers have alerted tranquilliser takers to the dangers of dependence, but because journalists have little real understanding of psychological problems, or of how drugs work, many people have been misled by sensational reporting and now feel not only frightened of becoming instantly addicted but also guilty about swallowing a tablet.

- A woman came to see me who was completely distraught and exhausted. Her child was very ill and she could not cope. People had told her that she should not use benzodiazepines, and she really came begging to me to sanction their use, which I did. She was desperate to have them sanctioned.

- In view of the recent publicity and criticism of doctors for putting half of the patients in the country on Valium I have made a much greater effort to resist prescribing it. But in the last couple of months I recollect two or three patients for whom I wanted to pre-scribe tranquillisers and who refused to have them.

Certainly, a large number of doctors have been too quick to reach for the prescription pad, but does this mean that these drugs should be banned altogether? Or can they sometimes play a part in dealing with emotional distress?

Most people who turn to their doctor when they are under stress feel better within a few weeks – whether they take tran-quillisers or not. After all, problems usually improve after a while and, if we have to learn to live with them, we need some time to adapt. But those who leave the surgery with a prescription in their pocket assume that it is the pills which have helped, and not that they would soon have felt better anyway. The next time they feel anxious they go back to the doctor, and each time this happens they are likely to take pills for longer than before.

● It is nice to give Valium for a week to a patient who has just been bereaved to help her sleep and calm her down. But often you end up with a patient who is on Valium for the rest of her life, especially if she is elderly. You start her on Valium at that time and she never stops taking it. It is very easy to use it, but very hard to stop.

Many people feel less anxious or depressed after taking a drug, not because of the chemicals in the drug, but simply because they have swallowed a tablet. We know that this is true because some people feel better even when they take a tablet which contains no drug at all. A fascinating experiment showed that people become either drowsy or alert, according to whether they are told the tablet they have taken is a depressant or a stimulant – even when the tablet contains no drug whatsoever! Not only does their behaviour alter, but physical changes in their body, such as pulse rate and blood pressure, also occur, rather as if they had taken the real drug. We are even affected by the appearance of the tablets we take, and coloured capsules are believed by their consumers to be better than white tablets, even when the drug in each is exactly the same.[16]

Learning to cope with any changes in our lives, whether they are for the better or the worse, can be stressful, and blotting out our feelings with pills can often prevent us from adjusting, rather than helping us to do so. But sometimes anxiety is so severe that we find ourselves trapped in a vicious circle – we are anxious because we are under stress, but we cannot deal with the stress because we are so anxious. When this happens, tranquillisers can help us break out of the trap – once we feel less anxious we become more able to cope, and because we can cope our anxiety decreases. Tranquillisers taken for a few weeks, and for this reason, will not cause dependence. In a similar way, anti-depressants can help break circles of deep depression.

Some people are more anxious than others when they are under stress and when these same people have particularly stressful lives they may feel anxious most of the time. If they decide to take tranquillisers for months or years they run the risk of dependence, and as time goes on this risk goes up while the effectiveness of the drugs goes down. Some long-term tranquilliser takers insist that their tablets still help them and protect them from a life of intolerable anxiety, and others manage to take them only when they need them, but most continue to take them, not because they feel better, but simply because they find it impossible to stop.

The problems so many people bring to their doctors cannot be removed by swallowing a pill. Rather than suppressing the symptoms of anxiety and depression with drugs, we need to find ways of removing the causes of emotional distress. Problems originating in society cannot be cured in the surgery. We need better child-care facilities, better housing, more jobs, improved laws about violence against women, and greater availability of counsellors and psychotherapists.

These are the ideal solutions to our problems, but where drugs are the only help offered to so many women, the decision to take them must be based on full knowledge of the risks involved.

The 1970s and 1980s have shown how women can influence doctors and how women can reassert control of their health. So far this has been mainly within obstetrics and gynaecology with women refusing to be treated as 'ill' when they are pregnant, refusing to lie on their backs in stirrups to give the doctor a better view when they are giving birth, insisting that birth is a normal process which in most cases they can control themselves by breathing, physical positions, help from fathers and friends and that they do not necessarily need drugs or intervention from doctors. The success of the women's movement in changing medical practices around reproduction has been impressively effective. It has spread to other areas like infertility, cervical smear tests, self-examination, support groups for mastectomy and hysterectomy patients and for rape victims.

It is time for this movement to assert women's control of their own psychological well-being: their minds, themselves. We can only begin to do this when we have a greater understanding of anxiety and depression, when we know the full effects of the drugs we may be offered, and when we are aware of the alternatives to drugs for coping with distress. With this knowledge we, and not only our doctors, can decide whether bottling it up is any answer to our emotional problems.

Part II Pills for our ills

6 Ill feelings

What is anxiety?[1,2]

Anxiety is unpleasant. It is like fear. Imagine you are in an aeroplane about to parachute for the first time: the ground looks a long way away and you are the next to jump. If you have that feeling when there is no immediate danger, that is anxiety.

Anxiety can range from a vague sense that something unpleasant is going to happen to an overwhelming attack of panic. Sometimes anxiety is thought of as an illness, and we are said to be 'suffering' from anxiety in the same way that we are said to be suffering from measles. There is no clear distinction, however, between this 'illness' and the familiar anxiety we experience when we find ourselves faced with a stressful or threatening situation. The difference is simply a matter of degree. Those diagnosed as suffering from anxiety tend to have these feelings more severely, for longer, and to such an extent that they interfere with everyday life. Some of us experience a single spell of anxiety, which lasts for a few days or weeks and then disappears, while others live in a recurring state of anxiety.

People who are anxious say they feel nervous, tense, uneasy, agitated, edgy and apprehensive, and often worry a lot. Their physical symptoms include a dry mouth, choking feelings, tense muscles, a tight or painful chest, rapid pounding of the heart, breathing difficulty, sweating, dizziness, light-headedness, shaking and the strange sensation of distance from the world.

- My heart starts to pound and an awful feeling of anxiety comes over me. I feel really scared. I am so dried up with nerves that even if someone was to offer me £1000 to spit I wouldn't be able to do it.

- I have tension in the back of my neck, tightness in my chest and palpitations. I cannot catch my breath and I shake all over.

These symptoms sometimes develop into an overpowering panic attack which makes people afraid of collapsing, fainting or a complete loss of control. A sudden urge to urinate, have a bowel movement, or be sick is not unusual.

- I feel fine one minute and then WHAM – I can't do anything. I shake, sweat, feel sick, my heart pounds and my legs are like jelly.

- I can't swallow and I feel as if my throat is closing up and that I shall choke. Panic washes over me and it is impossible to keep calm.

Insomnia is common during periods of anxiety, and when people do sleep they often have bad dreams. Tiredness and poor concentration can make getting through the day a huge effort, and bad temper develops for the most trivial reasons.

- I felt extremely tense and irritable, overwrought and tired. I wasn't sleeping. I became very irritable with the children and that is what made me go to the doctor.

Many people do not realise that these symptoms are caused by anxiety and may think that a thumping heart means they are about to have a heart attack, or that dizziness or light-headedness are signs of a brain tumour. This is hardly surprising but means that they feel even more anxious than before.

- If I had a pain I thought I had cancer or that I was going to have a heart attack. The slightest sore throat or indigestion made me think I had a serious illness. I blew every single minor pain out of proportion. I knew what I was doing but I couldn't control it.

What is a phobia?[3]

People who only become anxious in certain circumstances or when faced with something specific are said to have a phobia. They often go to great lengths to avoid whatever they fear, and even give up activities which they might otherwise enjoy. We probably all know of someone who would refuse the offer of an exciting trip abroad because of their fear of flying, but we might not be so familiar with those who stay indoors all summer because they are afraid of wasps and bees, or who turn down dinner invitations because the sight of a knife invokes instant terror. One woman we interviewed for this book took the stairs halfway up the tallest building in Britain to work every morning, and down again in the evening, rather than take the life.

Just think what it would be like to be afraid to go out, to travel on public transport, to visit your friends, to go shopping. That is what life is like for those who suffer from the most common phobia of all, agoraphobia.[4]

- Normal, everyday events like going to the shops or travelling any distance reduced me to a terrible state of nerves. Once, almost at the state of collapse, legs shaking, body trembling and feeling sick, I had to be brought home from work.

- I had a panic attack when I was at the supermarket queuing up to have my basket emptied. I thought 'I just have to get out of here.' I was trembling and my heart was pounding, and I felt that if I did not get out I would faint. It was really frightening, like something coming over me in a wave. I just had to get out of that store; I just wanted to run, I didn't know where but I couldn't stay where I was.

Many people with agoraphobia have to give up work and depend on others to do their shopping or any errand that involves going outside. They can become totally housebound unless they are accompanied by someone they know well.

They are not simply afraid of going out, but of having an anxiety attack if they do, and this has been described as suffering from a 'fear of fear'. A first reaction to panic is a desire to flee, so agoraphobics avoid places like shops and crowded buses where a quick exit may be impossible. Yet the more they avoid these places, the greater their fear of them. Unlike other phobias, it is not unusual for agoraphobia to be accompanied by general feelings of anxiety and depression.

Claustrophobia, the fear of enclosed spaces, is part of agoraphobia, but often occurs by itself.

- I am terrified by underground trains and by lifts and couldn't go in them on my own. If a lot of people come in I panic and just want to get out. I feel as if everything is closing in on me and I can't bear it.

Other phobias are of specific animals like cats or dogs, birds, snakes and, of course, the ubiquitous spider. Thunder and lightning, heights and darkness are also well-known phobias. Many of us fear the sight of blood and become very anxious about going to the doctor or dentist, especially if it involves having an injection. Some people are phobic about illness itself, imagining that the slightest pain or rash is the sign of a fatal disease, and in spite of their fear of all things medical they consult one doctor after another and endure endless tests in their never-ending search for reassurance.

The fear of social situations, known as social phobia, can be one of the most upsetting and cause acute isolation and loneliness. Afraid of what others might think of them, sufferers avoid mixing with people and are often particularly terrified of parties and public speaking.

- I lost my confidence and if anyone rang the bell I didn't want to open the door. I just didn't want to see anyone.

Like anxiety, a phobia is often mild enough to be kept under control and only becomes problematic when it interferes with everyday life. A petrifying fear, if we live in Britain, of koala bears will probably not prove too debilitating unless we have to earn our living by working in the animal house of our local zoo.

But a phobia which is so severe that it affects our family, social or working life can cause endless misery and should not be treated lightly.

What is depression?[5]

We all feel low and gloomy from time to time and say we are depressed. When these feelings take over and physical symptoms also develop we are said to have the 'illness' called depression. Like anxiety, there is no clear division between the mood and the 'illness'.

● I felt very low and very tearful. I started to get everything out of proportion and felt as if I couldn't cope. I found it very hard to snap out of it. I couldn't be bothered to talk to people. Everything was such an effort.

Depression can range from sadness and unhappiness to extreme misery and despair. People who are depressed cry easily, lose interest in others, and their work. Life seems boring and meaningless, and too much of an effort. Low self-confidence, poor concentration, and restlessness can make decisions or settling down to anything almost impossible. They often feel guilty and lose all sense of proportion about personal problems.

● I couldn't concentrate, I couldn't think and I couldn't do my job. I was unable to communicate with people or to follow a line of argument so I kept away from everyone at work. I lost all enjoyment in books and the theatre. I cried a lot and felt really awful.

● I had always been very bubbly and friendly but I became very quiet. I didn't have any interest in anything and I just wanted to stay at home. When my husband said, 'Let's go away for the weekend' or, 'We can pop over to France; it will give you a break' I just thought, 'Do we really have to?' It was too much of an effort. Nothing seemed exciting.

As depression sets in, the future appears hopeless and suicide can seem the only way out.

- I had this awful feeling to do away with myself. I didn't really want to do anything like that but the feeling just came over me. I took the overdose and thought I could just go and lie under a bush somewhere. It seemed the best solution. I thought I was going crazy and I didn't want people to say to my children, 'Your mum is in the looney bin'.

Insomnia, bad dreams and loss of appetite are common, although overeating is not unusual at first. Sufferers often complain of tiredness, lack of energy and a general slowing-down, as well as loss of interest in sex. Aches, pains, head-aches, a dry mouth, constipation, breathing problems and irritability can all occur with depression, and menstrual periods may become infrequent or even stop altogether.

- I feel as if I am fighting a battle with myself all the time to keep going. When I am at my worst I feel very low. I ask myself, 'What is the point of carrying on? Is it all worth it?' I just want to lie down and do nothing. I tell myself I am being stupid and that I should get up and do something but I do not seem to have the energy. I always feel so tired. I am only 61 years old but I feel like an old woman.

What is insomnia?[6]

Many people who are anxious or depressed complain that they cannot sleep. Those who are anxious are more likely to have trouble falling asleep, while those who are depressed often wake early in the morning or wake several times in the night and take a long time to fall asleep again. There are many poor sleepers who have no emotional problems at all, and although it is impossible to say exactly how many insomniacs there are, surveys show that up to 25 per cent of people over 30 years old have some difficulty in sleeping.

If we sleep badly we not only feel tired the next day, but are also unable to function well. There are no rules about how much sleep we should have to be at our best, and some people are quite happy with five or six hours a night while others say they need twice this amount. As we grow older we need less sleep, and people often worry about not sleeping enough simply because they sleep less than they used to, even although they feel no ill-effects the next day.

Do anxiety and depression run in families?[7,8]

We all know that children are sometimes very like other members of their family from an early age. In some cases the similarity between the personality of a small child and a grandfather or a great-aunt is striking in spite of the difference in age. People who adopt children and later meet the child's natural parents are often struck by their likeness in character although they have had no contact at all. An anxious or depressive predisposition may be inherited in the same way as other personality traits, but this does not mean that these people have something physically wrong with them or an 'abnormal' brain, or that they must be anxious or depressed throughout their lives. They may simply be more likely than others to develop anxiety or depression when they are under stress.

Another reason why anxiety and depression can run in families is that we imitate our parents. If our parents react to stress by becoming anxious or depressed, it is not surprising that we may learn to do the same, and people who are phobic have often grown up with a parent who becomes anxious in a similar situation. The way in which we deal with our emotional problems is obviously influenced by our parents.

● My mum is an anxious person and has been on pills for years, so
  when I became upset she took me to the doctor and he prescribed
  pills for me too. I was on them for 9 years. My mum has real faith
  in doctors and saw it all as natural.

81

But most of us with an anxious or depressed mother or father will not be anxious or depressed ourselves. There are many reasons why people have emotional problems, and passing them on from one generation to another is certainly not the only one.

What makes us anxious and depressed?

We are much more likely to become anxious and depressed if we are under stress. One of the most stressful experiences is the death of someone close to us, but problems in marriage, unemployment, poverty, poor housing, and growing older are others which can play havoc with our emotions.[9]

We may respond to stress by becoming either anxious or depressed. It is impossible to predict exactly how people will be affected, but depression is often connected to past events which have involved some kind of loss. Anxiety is more likely to be associated with fears about the future – not being able to pay our bills or the thought of a marriage breaking up. Someone who is anxious is also likely to feel depressed and vice versa.[10]

When people feel that they have some influence over the stress in their lives they are less vulnerable to its effects. As we saw in Part I, women often feel less in control of their lives than men and so are far more susceptible to depression and anxiety.[11]

What about physical causes?

The frequency with which people suffer depression after certain physical illnesses like influenza or glandular fever, and the fact that some people become severely depressed for no obvious reason, suggests that emotional problems may sometimes have biological causes, although exactly how this happens remains a mystery.[12]

Our bodies do affect our emotions, and many of us are familiar with the irritability, tiredness, poor concentration, tearfulness and feelings of anxiety and depression caused by premenstrual tension[13] and the menopause.[14] A few days after childbirth[15] more than 50 per cent of women experience the 'baby blues'. They become weepy for no apparent reason, and often feel anxious and worried about not being able to look after their baby. The 'baby blues' last only for a day or two. Postnatal depression affects only 10 per cent of mothers. It develops in the weeks after the baby is born, accompanied by anxiety about the child, irritability, exhaustion, insomnia and loss of appetite, although some women may overeat instead. The main concern of mothers experiencing postnatal depression is that they feel unable to cope, and often worry that there is something physically wrong with them. Postnatal depression which is so severe as to warrant admission to hospital is rare, and only happens to fewer than one in every 500 mothers. Women in this state are in such despair and misery that suicide, and sometimes even the death of their baby, can seem the only way out.

The hormones which cause the physical changes in women's bodies are often blamed for our emotional problems. Although this makes sense for premenstrual tension, depression after childbirth, and depression during the menopause, no one has actually proved it to be true. It seems likely that the emotional changes which take place at the same time as the changes in our bodies are just as much, if not more, to blame.

Why don't we all have emotional problems?

When we think of all the events in our lives which can lead to anxiety and depression, the question which comes to mind is not 'Why do people become anxious and depressed?' but instead 'How do some people seem to avoid it?' It is clear that the support of our family and friends is crucial for our emotional well-being, and if we do not have this support, we are much more likely to develop emotional problems.[16]

The success of the wide variety of groups which have been

set up so that people in similar circumstances can help each other, shows how social support makes a difference. As well as providing practical help the groups reduce feelings of isolation and loneliness, and people who join these groups in a state of desperation often find that within a few weeks they are giving as well as receiving help and advice. These groups have accomplished a great deal, but many of the people who might benefit feel too bad to make the effort to join one. After all, when life is getting on top of us the last thing we feel like doing is meeting new people.

An exciting project in the White City Estate in London has provided an answer to this dilemma. Women with emotional problems are given psychotherapy in their own neighbourhood and then, once they begin to feel better and ready to mix, they are also given the opportunity to help one another. Education groups have been set up to allow them to explore the connections between their social and emotional problems, and the effects of social issues on their everyday lives. The women are encouraged to examine both their past and present situations, and to find ways of improving their relationships and their environment. They are also put in touch with local individuals and organisations offering practical help, social contacts and support.

The result for many of these women has been a greater confidence, less anxiety and depression, and fewer tablets. The women no longer simply blame themselves for feeling unable to cope, which is a common response when we feel low. They have come to understand the effects of poor housing, financial hardship and lack of social support on their feelings, and together they have improved their lives on the estate.

There are thousands, like these women, struggling to look after their families without sufficient emotional, financial or practical support, and taking tranquillisers or antidepressants. The improvement in the emotional well-being of women involved in projects like the one at White City shows that confidence and the ability to cope cannot be chemically controlled.

7 Bitter pills

Psychotropic drugs are those drugs which act on the brain to alter our mood. This chapter will explain what they do to us and the differences between the drugs. The full effects of many of those which are commonly used are still being researched, but as we examine the opinions of both the women taking the drugs and the doctors prescribing them, the importance of current research will become clear.

Tranquillisers and sleeping pills

There are over 20 different kinds of benzodiazepines currently available in Britain and America – the most familiar and widely used are the tranquilliser diazepam (Valium) and the sleeping pill nitrazepam (Mogadon). Benzodiazepines are sold as either tranquillisers or sleeping pills but the effects of these drugs are so similar that a tranquilliser can be taken at night to help sleep, and a sleeping pill can be taken during the day to calm nerves. The different kinds of benzodiazepine drugs have to be taken in different amounts to have the same effect. For example, 1 milligram (mg) of lorazepam (Ativan) is equivalent to 5 milligrams (mg) of diazepam (Valium). Up to 3mg a day of lorazepam and 30mg a day diazepam are considered to be normal doses. Occasionally doctors prescribe drugs known as beta-blockers, like propranolol (Inderal), to calm us down. These are not tranquillisers, like benzodiazepines, but can reduce the physical symptoms of anxiety such as shaking and palpitations.

What effect do the various drugs have?
How do they differ?
Sleeping pills and tranquillisers differ from each other in the speed with which they have an effect. The length of time these drugs need to become effective depends on both the rate at which they are absorbed into the body, and how quickly they enter the brain. They can be divided into fast-acting and slow-acting pills. The sleeping pill nitrazepam is an example of a fast-acting drug which rapidly induces drowsiness. The tranquilliser lorazepam takes effect more quickly than diazepam and chlordiazepoxide (Librium) and is often prescribed for panic attacks.

Another difference between the various tranquillisers and sleeping pills is in the length of time they continue to have an effect once they begin to work. They can be divided into short-acting and long-acting pills. The tranquilliser lorazepam and the sleeping pill temazepam are short-acting drugs and disappear from the body fairly quickly once they have had an effect.

Tranquillisers like diazepam and chlordiazepoxide, and sleeping pills like nitrazepam are long-acting drugs and remain in the body for days. This is often considered to be beneficial in a tranquilliser as the drug continues to reduce anxiety between doses. Long-term accumulation is less desirable with sleeping tablets and doctors often recommend the short-acting brands as these overnight drugs should not cause sedation the following day.

When should I take the drugs and for how long?
Tranquillisers offer relief from anxiety in the first six weeks of a course of treatment. After this, there will be no marked changes: the drugs will maintain this level of improvement, but will not increase it.[1] The longer these drugs are taken on a *regular* basis, the less effective they become. Many of the thousands of people who have been taking pills on prescription for years are no longer benefiting from treatment – they are simply addicted.

In 1980 a report was published[2] which concluded that most sleeping pills lose their effectiveness within three to 14 days of continuous use, and after four months' steady intake of tranquillisers the pills may no longer reduce anxiety. Tranquillisers and sleeping pills can be effective over a longer period if they are *not* taken continuously, but *only* when we feel we need them. This may be once a month or once a week or for an entire week at irregular intervals. When taken in this way our bodies do not become so used to the drugs.

Shall I feel ill when I start taking the pills?
Side-effects[3] vary from person to person and they are most likely to occur during the first two weeks of a course of pills. The most common complaints are of drowsiness, lethargy and a feeling of heaviness as the smallest task becomes an enormous effort. Feelings of drowsiness will be at their worst within the first two hours of taking a tranquilliser during the day. If the sleeping pills are short-acting, there should be no after-effect in the morning, but this can be a problem with the long-acting variety. In addition, concentration and memory may be affected when first taking the pills.

If these side-effects occur it is advisable to put off important tasks or decisions, driving or working with mechanical and dangerous machinery for the first two weeks. Tranquillisers have been shown to affect driving and to increase the chance of accidents.

For some people, the drugs help them to think more clearly, as they counteract anxiety and exhaustion from lack of sleep. In rare cases, instead of having a calming effect, the drugs may cause an upsurge of the very symptoms they were prescribed to relieve. They can make people feel more anxious, sleep less well, have nightmares and cause emotional turmoil – weeping and giggling as well as hostility and aggression. In a few cases of shop-lifting and other crimes the defendants' behaviour has been explained by the fact that they were beginning a course of benzodiazepines, or taking an increased dose. These reactions are very rare, but can be extremely disturbing if the user does not see their connection to the particular drug they are taking.

After the first two weeks, the unwanted side-effects should wear off as our bodies have adjusted to the pills. They may not disappear completely but if there is little improvement of any kind the prescribed dose is probably too strong. Elderly people are particularly vulnerable when starting the pills and can become very confused while taking them.

Can I drink, or take other pills at the same time?
What happens when we mix tranquillisers or sleeping pills with alcohol is that the sedative effects of both are magnified. Drinking can be very dangerous while on a course of pills, and no one should drive after combining the two. One or two drinks are fairly safe as long as you know that it will slow down physical reactions and cause drowsiness, but it is best to avoid alcohol altogether while taking these drugs. Heavy drinking, or a high dose of diazepam or nitrazepam with a small amount of alcohol, can be fatal. It is safe to take other drugs while on sleeping pills or tranquillisers, but it is not advisable to mix them with other pills which cause drowsiness such as antidepressants or antihistamines as each will increase the other's sedative effect. If in doubt you should consult your doctor before taking any other drugs.

It is very important to recognise the potential hazards of these drugs when they are first prescribed. As women are the biggest consumers of tranquillisers and sleeping pills they also form the majority of overdose victims. It is rare that an overdose of benzodiazepines alone proves fatal, but it is possible. Usually the overdose causes a deep sleep lasting for one or two days. The combination of tranquillisers or sleeping pills and alcohol or other drugs is the commonest cause of overdose in America, and is often fatal. It is tragic that so often these are accidental suicides which could have been avoided if the women had known more about the drugs they were taking.

What are the long-term effects?
These were the comments of women who had been on tranquillisers for a long period.

- I had no concentration. I couldn't remember anything, even my own phone number. My emotions were all on one level. I didn't appreciate life.
- My memory was awful. I couldn't make a decision and stick to it.
- My head felt fuzzy.
- I felt as if I was doped. I remember going shopping one day, getting off the bus and completely forgetting what I had wanted to buy.
- I felt like a robot.
- I didn't notice anything around me. The colours of the flowers or the birds singing.
- After two or three years I realised I wasn't living. I was just existing. I felt as if I was drugged all the time.

At the moment, research into the long-term effects of tranquillisers and sleeping pills is still in its early stages. While we know a great deal about the initial effects of these drugs it is vital that we discover much more about their continuous use over long periods.

If I become pregnant, will the drugs affect my baby?
Many women are told not to take drugs while they are pregnant, but few know what might happen if they do because there are no definite answers to this question, and much of the evidence to support the view that tranquillisers taken during early pregnancy produce malformed babies is inconclusive.[4] We do know, however, that the large majority of mothers who have taken tranquillisers during the early stages of pregnancy have had normal babies – so the risk appears to be very low. Some investigations show that cleft lips and cleft palates may be more common among babies whose mothers have been on tranquillisers during the first three months of pregnancy but evidence is inconclusive.

There is far more known about the harmful effects of these drugs when taken during late pregnancy, but such effects do not always occur. They can intoxicate the baby causing 'the floppy infant syndrome'. This means that newborn babies are unable to suck properly and have difficulty breathing and feeding. The higher the dose taken by the mother, the more severe will be the baby's symptoms, but even small doses taken repeatedly may have this effect. If tranquillisers are taken continuously for several months in late pregnancy, the infant may suffer withdrawal symptoms a few hours after delivery. These can last for several weeks, and most commonly produce trembling and difficulty with feeding and digestion.

If the mother is taking drugs while breast-feeding, they will be absorbed straight into the milk and may affect the baby with lethargy and weight loss. The *British National Formulary* recommends that tranquillisers and sleeping pills should be avoided if at all possible during breast-feeding.

Are tranquillisers and sleeping pills addictive?

Benzodiazepines taken in high doses were reported to be addictive when they first appeared in the 1960s. Recent investigations have carefully monitored what happens to people when they stop taking normal amounts of these prescribed drugs and provide clear evidence that the drugs *are* addictive.[5,6] It has taken the medical profession 20 years to begin to acknowledge this danger. The medical journals, which represent the profession's views and keep most doctors in touch with developments, have disclaimed that sleeping pills and tranquillisers are addictive: 'While psychological and physical dependence on benzodiazepines may occur, this is rare and is not cause for alarm.' (*Journal of the American Medical Association*, 1979.)

Addicts certainly do exist in large numbers, but few of them have been recognised, let alone reported, by the medical profession itself. In 1978 a survey of all published reports of benzodiazepine dependence implied that less than 500 people in the entire world had ever become addicted. This kind of material helps doctors to believe in the truth of their training – that these drugs are not addictive.[7] It is only in the face of incontrovertible evidence from Britain and America that the most widely read medical journal in Britain has begun to indicate a change of heart: 'Several investigations ... have shown quite unequivocally that benzodiazepines may produce pharmacological dependence in therapeutic dosage'. (*British Medical Journal*, 1984.)

Why has it taken so long for the danger of addiction to be acknowledged? Is it purely because it is against the doctors' interests to have to stop prescribing these drugs? Or are there medical grounds for their reticence?

What makes an addict?
One reason that doctors rarely recognise addiction to such drugs is because these pill-poppers do not show the same signs as other drug addicts. To most doctors an addict is someone whose dependency on a drug means that the dose has to be increased for it to continue to take effect, and who will go to any length to keep up the supply. This classic pattern fits only a tiny minority of benzodiazepine addicts. Most will remain on the dose which the doctor has prescribed, or even manage to reduce it after a while and continue at a lower level. Those who increase their dose usually do so only when life becomes particularly stressful, and cut down again when problems ease.

People who find themselves addicted to tranquillisers or sleeping pills may not recognise their own condition. Once prescribed, these pills are easy to obtain and repeat prescriptions are often given without question. If one doctor should refuse, there will always be another who will comply, or friends and relatives with an immediate supply.

Another sign of addiction is a withdrawal effect when the pills are stopped. In the case of tranquillisers and sleeping pills this often includes anxiety and insomnia, so it is not surprising that doctors often fail to recognise addiction. They assume these symptoms to be a return of the original problem and prescribe more tranquillisers and sleeping pills.

- I stopped my pills from time to time and had withdrawal symptoms, but I didn't know what they were. I thought I had a physical illness. I didn't connect the symptoms with the tablets. I saw a physician; he said there was nothing physically wrong with me. He prescribed more tranquillisers. They made me feel better but I was back to square one.

- I was told I had blocked sinuses. I went to an ear, nose and throat specialist. He said I was over-breathing and prescribed tranquillisers. I went back on them. It had been very hard to come off them but I felt so low.

A matter of facts – addiction and withdrawal

In Britain alone there are approximately 250 000 benzodiazepine addicts, and in America 1 000 000. One in every three people who take tranquillisers and sleeping pills continuously for more than six months will have withdrawal symptoms when they stop. Not everyone has problems coming off these drugs, and we do not know why some people are affected while others are not.

We do know that the longer these drugs are taken on a regular basis, the more likely it is that dependence will occur. Withdrawal symptoms can appear after as little as four months on a particular drug, and with short-acting pills this can happen even earlier – the tranquilliser lorazepam (Ativan) is especially difficult to come off and causes more cases of addiction than other pills. A low dose of a drug does not mean that the withdrawal symptoms will be fewer or less severe. Most people become dependent on the normal dose prescribed by their doctor, and although higher doses carry greater risks, withdrawal symptoms can be just as unpleasant whether they result from a high or low intake of the drugs.

Experiences of withdrawal
As it takes time for the drugs to disappear from the body, withdrawal symptoms will not occur immediately after stop-

ping the tablets or decreasing the dose. With short-acting drugs like lorazepam, they may take effect within one day, but with the longer-acting ones, like diazepam, it is usually a couple of days or even a week before symptoms develop. Symptoms are often at their worst after a week without drugs and can disappear within a month, but they may persist for up to a year before they finally disappear.[8,9]

- I began to feel as though I was tottering. It was like having had a crutch for years and finally I was walking without any aid at all. I felt very insecure. I didn't know what was happening to me. Nobody told me. That was the most frightening part. Not knowing what was happening to me.

As with side-effects, withdrawal symptoms vary from person to person. The most common and often the first to occur are anxiety and insomnia – the very symptoms the drugs were prescribed to cure.

- I had insomnia all through this period. I just didn't sleep at all.
- I felt dizzy, my legs were shaking, I felt as if I wasn't here. I was so panicky inside about something but I didn't know what it was. I couldn't breathe.

As well as feelings of nervousness and tension the physical symptoms of anxiety such as sweating, palpitations, choking feelings, dizziness and shaking can appear. These can develop into an overwhelming panic attack.

- I was perspiring all over. My hands were shaking.
- I used to sit in the corner of the room and just shake and sweat continuously.
- The palpitations at night were the worst symptoms. I thought something was going to explode. I felt my heart couldn't keep beating like that without something terrible happening. I was dead tired and wanted to go to sleep but I couldn't. I would lie there and feel the thumping in my chest. It felt as though the whole room was echoing with my heartbeat. Those were the most frightening periods.

It is not unusual for people to fear leaving the house.

- I lost my confidence. I wanted to crawl back and hide.

- When I went into a shop I felt closed in and had to rush out and get home quickly, legs shaking, panic taking over me, battling with my mind to keep calm.

Many people experience the peculiar sensation of distance from the world.

- I felt as if my mind was outside my body, as if my mind was over there and my body was here. It was a terrible feeling.

- I felt as if I was in a plastic bubble. I felt more and more isolated and withdrawn.

Concentration and memory can be affected and there is loss of energy.

- I was driving the car and literally didn't know what I was doing. It was as if I didn't know how to drive or as if someone else was driving the car.

- I didn't dress and I didn't wash for a week. I just sat in a chair.

Often people going through withdrawal feel as if they have flu. Some people lose their appetite, feel nauseous and may be sick, while others suffer dreadful hunger. Constipation, diarrhoea, headaches, muscle aches and pains often develop. Muscles can even twitch and jerk quite dramatically.

- I am going through withdrawal at the moment. My whole body aches, I am physically sick and my head feels as if it is in a vice.

- I was sick. I was incontinent. I had this dreadful head.

- I had intense hunger. I couldn't stop eating. I ate and drank at about half-hour intervals for four days but I wasn't full up. It was like trying to fill up a sink with no plug in it.

- It was like very bad flu which never goes away.

Some people feel depressed as well as anxious.

- I cried continuously.

- It affected me emotionally, I was very weepy. Sudden, uncontrollable weeping for no apparent reason would strike me in the most unexpected places, at home, at my office and even while out socially. I was very unsure of myself. My confidence went totally.

- I had this awful feeling to do away with myself, yet I didn't want to do anything like that, but that was just the feeling that came over me.

Blurred or double vision, and acute sensitivity or numbness can be part of withdrawal. Bright lights and loud noises can become unbearable, and sometimes unusual smells and tastes are noticed.

- I went through a period of awareness as though I was seeing and hearing things for the first time. All my senses were accentuated. Everything seemed extra bright and extra loud. Colours were very bright. The birds seemed not to be singing but bellowing.

- As I got up in the morning pins and needles began at the tips of my fingers and then travelled up my wrists, up my arms and then over my entire body. I was a mass of pins and needles and numbness.

- I was very giddy. My body felt pulled to the left side.

- My vision was affected. It was like looking through watery eyes. This lasted for several weeks. I kept looking at the trees to see if they were still blurred.

In very rare instances the symptoms of withdrawal may cause fits, severe confusion and the type of mental illness known as psychosis, which causes people to lose touch with reality and behave in a bizarre fashion. Those suffering from a pyschotic reaction may hear voices, or see things which do not actually exist.

- I went through a terrible stage of confusion. I made a journey on the Tube. It was a route I knew very well. When I had to change platforms I didn't know whether to turn left or right. I was confused by a simple thing like changing platforms in a railway station. Familiar places seemed almost alien to me. It was a very strange sensation, a feeling of being lost.

- I had hallucinations and kept screaming during the night.

Staying power

Some people suffer so badly when they try to stop taking benzodiazepines that they feel totally discouraged. When withdrawal sets in, staying on the tablets can seem preferable to the nightmare of trying to come off.

- I have been taking Valium for 15 years. I have tried to give them up many times but after a few days I feel upside down.
- In the past 10 years I have had a few short spells off Valium. When I stop them I don't notice for a day or two but after a week I feel awful. I always end up back at the surgery.

Others, who manage to struggle through, feel that coming off benzodiazepines was one of the worst experiences they have ever had.

- I'll never forget it in my whole life. I thought I was going to die. I thought I was going to crack up. I thought I was going insane.

Lack of support from family and friends can make matters worse.

- My husband got fed up with it all. He thought I should just throw the pills in the dustbin and get on with it. He said that all I needed was will-power. I had no support, which was so hard.

But not everyone has trouble in stopping.

- I was taking three 15mg Librium a day. It was my own decision to stop. For a while I had two each day, then one, and then I gradually didn't have any. It took me a couple of months to come off them but I didn't find it difficult.

It is easier to cut down the pills gradually than to stop suddenly.

96

- I saw a television programme about the effects of tranquillisers. I didn't like the fact that I was addicted and decided to stop Valium dead. I felt uptight and awful and had incredible panics. I tried to combat it but couldn't. After a few days I ended up popping a pill. That calmed me down. I thought 'thank God that is over'.

But reducing gradually doesn't always mean that it won't be difficult. It can take months and sometimes more than a year. Symptoms can come and go long after stopping the tablets.

- It took me a year to get the symptoms out of my body. Each time I cut down another half tablet I had six days of really bad symptoms before they began to wear off. I had to wait for weeks on end to feel normal again.

- I took my last tablet over four months ago. It has not been easy and still isn't at times. But now, when I get these awful feelings, I know they will go away.

- I had my last tablet one and a half years ago. It took nearly a year to feel back to normal. It seemed so very slow, as if I was never going to get better. Only by looking back could I see any improvement.

Sometimes the last step is the worst.

- I was petrified of letting go of the last half tablet. I kept thinking 'How am I going to cope without a pill? How can I go out any more?' The withdrawal symptoms were at their worst at this stage. I tried and tried to get off, but I couldn't do it.

- I reduced my daily dose by 1mg of Valium at a time. I got down from 30mg a day to 6mg a day. Then I don't know what happened. I had a terrible bout of nerves. I thought I was going raving mad. I thought I had flipped.

Is it all worth it?

- I felt very vulnerable after I stopped: as if my protection had been ripped away; as if I was walking about naked. I wasn't used to dealing with my emotions. It was like coming out a dark wine bar at lunchtime into the bright street. But I felt more alive. It was like being reborn. It was the first spring I was aware of for years. My senses were waking up again. I was more aware of the flowers and the trees.

● I was on Valium for 15 years. Since I have been off I feel much better. I have confidence. I feel it is my own confidence. Before, I knew it was only the pills which gave me confidence. Now when I get up in the morning I don't need anything to make me go out and do things. I feel like I used to before I started the tablets. For years I never used to notice the colour of the grass or the birds. Now I notice these things just like when I used to live in the country. I walk along and think that the birds sound lovely. When I was on the tablets I just used to go on from day to day without noticing things around me. I feel that I wasted all these years on tablets. I never wanted to go out. Now I go out all the time. I feel I have missed out on a lot. I have just started decorating, which I would never have had the confidence to do before. I notice a big difference. I feel alive again.

Antidepressants

Antidepressants are sometimes taken for long periods of time, and, although they are not generally thought to be addictive, some concern is now growing that people do have trouble in stopping. The most commonly prescribed antidepressants belong to the group of drugs called tricyclics, such as amitriptyline (Tryptizol) and imipramine (Tofranil).[10] These can help relieve depression but do not work for 30 per cent of people who take them. It is impossible to predict precisely who will benefit, but these antidepressants are thought to be more effective for people who not only feel depressed but who also have the physical symptoms of depression, such as loss of appetite and insomnia. Some doctors believe that these drugs are more likely to help people who are depressed for no clear reason, rather than because of a specific event in their lives.

Antidepressants only work if the correct dose is taken. Often people try to take as low a dose of a drug as possible, and although this may be sensible with tranquillisers, antidepressants will have no effect at all. Often it is two to three weeks before they begin to take effect. Initially, people feel worse rather than better, adding unpleasant side-effects to the depression. When this happens, many give up and either stop the pills altogether, or decrease their dose to an ineffectual level.

When antidepressants do work, improved sleep and a healthier appetite are often the first noticeable benefits. Gradually, energy returns and feelings of depression begin to lift. Most people who are helped by these drugs feel less depressed after a month or six weeks, but they are usually advised to keep taking the pills for at least three months, and often much longer if they have been depressed in the past, to lessen their chances of becoming depressed again. In the process of coming off antidepressants, the dose should be reduced gradually to minimise side-effects and to make sure that depression is not returning.

Different antidepressants vary in their chemical structure and effect, and everyone will have different reactions. If a particular drug is not working after a month or so, a change of drug may well help. Some cause more drowsiness than others, and people suffering from depression and anxiety may benefit more from the sedative types of drug. Those who already feel lethargic may prefer the less sedative kind.

What are the side-effects?
Side-effects[11] are quite common and often unpleasant. They may develop after only one pill, or within a few days. As the body adjusts to the drugs, the side-effects diminish, and once the depression begins to lift the side-effects are easier to bear.

The most common side-effects are a dry mouth, blurred vision and constipation. They may cause drowsiness or, in some cases, insomnia. The whole dose for each 24 hours can sometimes be taken at night and this can help insomnia and lessen drowsiness during the day. Like tranquillisers and sleeping pills, they can affect clear thinking and no one should drive or operate dangerous machinery when beginning the pills. Sweating, trembling, difficulty in passing water and light-headedness may occur. The drugs can cause an increase in appetite, particularly for sweet and starchy foods, and people who take antidepressants often complain of putting on weight. Occasionally sexual problems develop and men may complain of not having erections or of taking a long time to ejaculate, while women may find difficulty reaching orgasm.

Antidepressants can be dangerous to anyone with a heart disease, by speeding up the heartbeat and making the rhythm irregular. Occasionally, these drugs lead to glaucoma and epileptic fits, particularly if a user has a history of such problems. The elderly tend to have more severe side-effects and can become extremely confused or delirious.

Can I take other drugs while on antidepressants?

Mixing drugs can be very dangerous and even fatal. No other medicines of any kind should be taken with antidepressants without consulting a doctor. This is true even of drugs which can be bought without a prescription, such as antihistamines and medicines for the common cold. It is not safe to drink alcohol while on a course of tricyclics as this mixture increases the sedative effects of both drugs.

As many as 10 per cent of drug-overdose suicides use tricyclics. The most common result of an overdose is coma, and death can be caused by heart failure, breathing problems, or convulsions.

Is my baby in danger if I become pregnant?

In the early 1970s an Australian medical journal published an article warning that if a pregnant woman took tricyclics she ran the risk of giving birth to a deformed baby. This report was later shown to be unfounded, but it triggered off a number of investigations all over the world.[see 4] The Australian Drug Evaluation Committee concluded: 'available information does not support the contention that tricyclic antidepressants are a cause of limb-reduction deformities'. If these drugs, however, are taken in late pregnancy, the newborn baby may temporarily have a rapid heartbeat, breathing difficulties and muscle spasms. Tricyclics are only absorbed into the mother's milk in very small quantities and have not been found to harm the baby.

New developments

In recent years new antidepressants have been developed in an attempt to overcome the disadvantages of the older ones. So far this has not produced a more effective alternative, but it has led to drugs with less unpleasant side-effects.[12] These are often prescribed for the elderly and are less likely to be fatal if taken in overdose.

One of the latest offerings is a drug advertised for use in 'anxiety associated with depression'. Although the company which produces this drug is careful not to describe it as a drug which relieves both anxiety *and* depression, this is just how some doctors see it.

- I tend to prescribe this drug. It is supposed to relieve anxiety and depression and since the two are so linked together I think it is a good drug.

- Now the drug companies have brought out a new drug which is partly for anxiety and partly for depression, but I am a bit doubtful about it. A drug that will treat both anxiety and depression is like a pig in a poke. If you do not know which drug to give, then give this one because it does both.

Even if this drug was to live up to its reputation, pills rarely provide the best long-term solution. The next chapter offers some alternative ways of coping with emotional problems.

Part III Coming off and coping

8   Alternatives

Most people need help in coming off pills and coping with life without them. What kinds of help are available? In this chapter we shall look at different types of therapy offered by psychologists, psychoanalysts and counsellors, at techniques for relaxing physical tension, at some forms of alternative health care, and at self-help groups.

None of the alternatives is as effortless as swallowing a pill. It is not a question of simply switching from your doctor to a psychologist or a homoeopath and receiving a 'substitute' for your pills. Rather it is a matter of learning how your lifestyle affects your health and how you can cope with stress, depression or anxiety without drugs.

Some doctors are themselves trying to help provide their patients with alternatives by involving psychologists in group practices or by working in close liaison with health visitors, social workers, and some volunteer organisations. Other doctors are active in community projects and local support groups on issues like housing, child care facilities and provision for the elderly. Increasingly, GPs are encouraging patients with similar problems to get together in self-help groups. The majority of people, however, will still find few, if any, alternatives easily available in the surgery.

Seeing a therapist

There are many different therapies for emotional problems which have one thing in common – they consider emotional problems to arise from experiences in our lives rather than chemicals in our bodies. Even when the cause of our problems may be partly physical, they still try to make sense of, and deal with, our experiences. The main types of therapy which you are likely to be offered if you go to a psychologist or a psychiatrist fall under the headings below,[1] and some specific techniques are described in more detail in the self-help withdrawal programme.

The main difference between a psychologist and a psychiatrist is that a psychiatrist is medically qualified and can prescribe drugs. Many psychiatrists, like psychologists, offer therapy to their patients, but others are more likely to write a prescription. Other people may also train as therapists and the word 'psychotherapist' can be used to describe a therapist of any kind.

Not everyone finds therapy helpful, but many people do. A group of researchers found that emotionally distressed people who saw a psychologist, rather than a doctor, not only felt better more quickly but also took fewer drugs, and the amount of money that was saved on drugs was enough to pay for 28 per cent of the psychologist's salary![2]

Relaxation therapy[3]

One of the most widely used therapies for anxiety is relaxation, which makes sense because it is impossible to be both anxious and relaxed at the same time. The technique of deep muscle relaxation has been used in therapy to help relieve anxiety since the 1930s, and there are many other variations such as hypnotherapy and meditation. Relaxation therapies focus mainly on the physical symptoms of anxiety. The self-help guide tells you how to teach yourself relaxation therapy.

Behaviour therapy[4]

Behaviour therapy concentrates on changing behaviour, and it works well for phobias. If we become frightened in a certain situation and then begin to avoid that situation because we are afraid, we fear it even more. Unless we give ourselves the chance to experience that same situation when we are not afraid, we may never get rid of our fear. So, if someone in a boat is frightened by a rough sea, the next time a friend suggests a sail she may feel too nervous to accept in case a storm brews up. If she stops sailing altogether, her fear will persist and may lead to a permanent phobia. Alternatively, if she goes sailing again and again, and experiences no more stormy seas, her fear will die away.

Therapy is usually directed towards helping people gradually to get used to whatever it is they fear. Sometimes this is done by imagining the frightening situation while deeply relaxed, but often it involves approaching it in real life.

Behaviour therapists believe that people become depressed because their lives are not rewarding, and that people who do not feel in control of what happens to them are particularly vulnerable. Behaviour therapy for depression concentrates on helping people to make their lives more satisfying by training them in coping skills and in how best to go about solving their problems.

Cognitive therapy[5,6]

Cognitive therapy has become popular in recent years as a way of dealing with anxious thoughts and worries. People are encouraged to recognise their anxious thoughts, for example, 'I cannot cope', and to substitute more useful ones, like 'I can try it one step at a time'. When we are anxious we tend to think in an irrational and illogical way. Cognitive therapy helps people to understand how anxiety distorts the way they interpret and react to situations, and to see these situations more realistically.

Cognitive therapists also help people to change the negative attitudes and false beliefs which make them feel depressed. When we feel low we are likely to get things out of proportion, or jump to conclusions without enough evidence. So if a friend does not ring up as arranged, someone who is depressed will probably think, 'She does not like me any more', rather than, 'Perhaps she was busy, or could not get to a telephone', and end up feeling even more depressed. Therapy concentrates on helping people to identify their negative thoughts, to consider alternative viewpoints, and to test them out.

Psychoanalysis[7]

Psychoanalysts believe that emotional problems can stem from unpleasant past experiences which have been locked away in the unconscious mind. They help their patients to explore these unconscious feelings so that they may gain a better understanding of their present problems and relationships in the light of their past. This understanding develops through the evolving therapeutic relationship between the patient and the analyst. The patient develops strong feelings for the analyst which allow the patient to re-experience childhood emotions and thus come to terms with them. With full psychoanalysis the client attends a 50-minute therapy session five days a week for several years. The therapy involves lying on a couch and talking freely about whatever comes to mind.

Psychoanalytic psychotherapy is more common than full psychoanalysis. It is based on the psychoanalytic approach, but the client attends therapy only once or twice a week for a shorter period of time and does not lie on a couch. Therapy is concerned with specific psychological problems and, like traditional psychoanalysis, examines the connections between present experiences and past events.

Counselling[8]

Counselling gives people the opportunity to talk about their problems. The client is in control of what is discussed, and by listening, asking questions, and trying to understand what is being said, the counsellor helps the client to work out ways of dealing with difficulties. The counsellor is not judgemental and tries to create an atmosphere which will help the client to talk freely. Counsellors often specialise in particular kinds of problems, like marital problems or abortion.

Marital therapy, sex therapy and family therapy[9,10,11]

Marital therapy can help couples who are distressed about their relationship and who feel they are unable to solve their problems themselves. They do not have to be married, but they must both take part. Common problems revolve around the fact that one or both partners feel that the other is hostile, dominating or not close enough. Therapy is usually aimed at making the relationship more satisfying, but sometimes the couple are helped to decide to separate instead. Some marital therapists help the couple to learn how to communicate better, how to solve their problems more effectively, and how to get what they want out of the relationship by giving in return. Others concentrate more on reorganising the relationship by helping the couple to see their problems from a different point of view, and to recognise how their ways of doing things can lead to problems.

Couples who have sex therapy complain often of a general lack of interest or enjoyment in sex, but sometimes their problems are more specific. Common problems for men are impotence and premature ejaculation. Women may be concerned about not feeling aroused, or not having an orgasm, and some find that their vaginal muscles go into a spasm which makes them unable to have intercourse. Therapy involves the couple carrying out a series of exercises at home which are aimed at helping them to feel more relaxed, to communicate about their sexual relationship and to deal with their problem in a systematic way. When they see the therapist they discuss their progress, as well as how to deal with any difficulties which have cropped up. The therapist also suggests specific techniques which might help them.

Family therapists deal with emotional problems by involving the whole family in therapy. So, if an individual is depressed, they would explore how relationships among family members might contribute to that person's depression. They try to alter family relationships by focusing on patterns of communication, how decisions are made, who are the dominant members, which roles are performed by whom, and alliances among family members.

Therapy can help women to understand their problems and change their lives in a positive way. It can reduce anxiety and depression, and enable them to cope with their difficulties. There is no single type of therapy which is more effective than others; different people will feel comfortable with different approaches. But therapy has its limitations. It deals only with the experiences of an individual person, an individual couple, or an individual family, and does little to change the social disadvantage and inequality which are so often responsible for women's problems in the first place. Often therapy is aimed at helping women adjust to their situation, rather than improve it. In recent years there has been a move towards a better understanding of women's problems and services have been set up to cater specifically for women's needs.

The importance of what we eat and drink

● I saw one woman last week who was taking nitrazepam [sleeping pills]. She was drinking about 10 cups of coffee a day and didn't bother to eat breakfast because she was so hyped up for work in the morning she didn't have time. For lunch it was something quick like a sandwich and then rushing home and having instant supper from tins or packets. It's not surprising she had sleeping problems. I always start by trying to change people's attitudes to what they are putting inside their bodies.

Coffee and tea contain caffeine. Caffeine is a stimulant drug which in high doses makes people anxious. So caffeine and tranquillisers are opposites. If you are cutting down tranquillisers or sleeping pills, it is wise to cut down coffee and tea as well, otherwise you will feel more anxious and have more sleep difficulties than you need to. Try drinking water, fruit juice, herbal teas or decaffeinated coffee instead.

Even though many of us drink alcohol to feel 'merry' or 'high', it is a depressant drug which, if you are already feeling

110

down, will only make you feel worse. Alcohol is often used as a 'night-cap' to help people sleep better. Although you might fall asleep faster after drinking, the effects are short-lived and sleep during the second half of the night is often broken. So alcohol does not work well as a sleeping potion. Again, many people drink to help them relax when they are tense or worried. This is fine from time to time, but used a lot and regularly it can cause dependence on alcohol, with disastrous results.

We know less about the effects of different foods on feelings of anxiety and depression. There are cases of children who have been labelled hyperactive, given tranquillisers and subsequently found to have been allergic to a particular food. Refined sugar has also been implicated as a factor in depression and in migraine.[12] Often we do not really know what we are eating and it comes as a shock to read the list of ingredients on tins, jars, bottles and packets. Mary found changing her diet helped her when she was coming off tranquillisers:

● I went on a wholemeal diet when I was coming off. I drank lots of orange juice and things with vitamin C. And I ate plenty of fresh vegetables every day. The homoeopathic doctor gave me tablets made only from vegetables, which contained vitamin B. I felt so well on the diet. It was pretty expensive but it really helped and did me the world of good.

A healthy diet normally contains all the vitamins we need, but some women do find supplements of vitamin B help, especially with premenstrual tension and nerves.

Exercise

Many women find exercise helpful. Working your body helps relieve the physical tension in muscles, helps get you going when you feel lifeless, and often means you sleep better. Exercise does not have to mean aerobics or jogging round the

111

park. A brisk walk instead of taking the bus to work, a swim, gardening, climbing the stairs instead of taking the lift; there are lots of ways of making a bit of extra physical effort. It is important to exercise gradually, starting in a small way and building up a little more over a period of time.

Yoga

Yoga is helpful for tension and stress because it combines the advantages of exercise on the one hand with those of mental relaxation (through meditation) on the other. It is suitable for people of all ages and it can be very helpful during pregnancy. Yoga classes can usually be found locally and are generally inexpensive.

The Alexander principle

The Alexander principle is a therapy which aims to treat and prevent a range of disorders by a system of changes in posture. Over the years, many people have developed habits of slouching, slumping and tensing-up muscles. A teacher of the Alexander principle will assess problems with your posture, not just how you stand but how you sit, lie and so on. She will then show you how to correct your posture, how to relax the tension in your body and, according to your individual needs, give you a series of exercises you can do at home.

● My Alexander teacher showed me how to recognise when I was physically tense and how to relax. Relaxing physically also made me relax mentally so it really was my mainstay when I came off tranquillisers. I've used it ever since.

The number of lessons you need depends on you. Some people finish the course after 12 lessons, others need many more. It is an especially useful technique to learn if anxiety is associated with pains in the back or with general physical tension.

Alternative medicine[13]

There are now many forms of health care available outside orthodox medical care. Once dismissed as the 'lunatic fringe' of medicine, acupuncture, homoeopathy, herbalism and other alternatives are now receiving renewed attention, especially for problems for which orthodox medicine has not been able to offer solutions. As yet there is little scientific evaluation of alternative health care and there are many 'quacks' around who are untrained.

Different forms of alternative medicine have certain ideas in common. First, they all believe in treating the person as a whole, looking not only at your physical symptoms but at your lifestyle: what you eat, how you exercise, what stresses and strains you have at home and at work. Although orthodox medicine may agree with holistic principles that social and emotional factors affect our physical and mental 'health', not many doctors have time to counsel their patients about diet, exercise or stress.

- Within the perspective of any holistic medicine, a symptom is exactly that – it's a symptom *of* something, a warning light that something is going wrong somewhere. The mistake orthodox medicine often makes is to think that the symptoms – say the depression or insomnia – are the actual problem. They are not. One needs to deal with the underlying problems. (An acupuncturist.)

- You are really treating a whole person and not just using herbalism or any other holistic medicine as symptomatic relief. You look at all points of the triangle – physical, social and environmental factors – to work out which factors are influencing which parts of the body. (A herbalist.)

So people cannot expect to go to someone practising alternative medicine and be given an 'alternative' pill to a tranquilliser or antidepressant.

- Quite a lot of patients who are taking sleeping pills or tranquil-lisers come to me and expect me to give them a homoeopathic pill which they can just put in their place. It's not like that, we don't just treat symptoms. (A homoeopath.)

- I see acupuncture like any other proper form of health care, as actually trying to hand the capacity for health back to the person. It's to do with advising and helping the person to become aware of what it is in their lives that is making them ill and what they can do about it. One could do this within orthodox medicine but not with the high turnover rate perpetuated by orthodox doctors. (An acu-puncturist.)

Part of the reason some people are helped by alternative medicine is that they are given a lot of time to talk and they are listened to. So, for some people, the effectiveness of alternative medicine may be due more to the emotional sup-port and 'counselling' they receive than to the 'treatments' they are given. Whether or not the 'treatments' actually work remains an open question. Very few objective studies have been carried out and there is no scientific evidence as yet that alternative treatments are any more effective than giving a harmless placebo. Further, any treatment – be it orthodox or alternative – which is aimed at correcting 'imbalances' in the individual cannot begin to solve social causes of anxiety and depression.

Acupuncture

- We never start by saying, 'Right, you have got to give up these drugs', whatever those drugs are, or this or that junk food or any-thing else to do with a person's life. But by working with people, it generally comes from them; it's the person who tells me, 'Hey! I want to get off these drugs', or asks me, 'Should I stop eating all that rubbish?' or, 'Should I start doing this or that?' It's at that point one can actually work with the person and help them move through the process. I think a step-down approach is advisable with almost any drugs, reducing them bit by bit.

What happens when you go to an acupuncturist for the first time?

114

- We start by listening to the person most of the time. A lot of it can be counselling. I allow up to two hours for the first session when, through learning about the person, I build up a diagnosis. After the first session it's usually one-hour treatments.

The diagnosis is based on what has been learnt about the client's case history, lifestyle, habits, and so on, and also on a physical examination which starts with taking six 'pulses' on each wrist and examining the tongue. The acupuncturist will discuss the diagnosis with the client and agree on a course of action and treatment.

Treatment will consist mainly of inserting very fine needles into appropriate points along 'meridians' and the aim is to correct the diagnosed 'imbalances' in the body. Other forms of treatment include moxibustion – applying heat to the appropriate acupuncture points.

Herbalism
Orthodox medicine originated in herbalism, where natural herbs are used to heal and strengthen the mind and body. Fifty years ago, some herbal preparations, such as extract of dandelion, were still marketed by drug companies.

The first time you visit a herbalist, the main concern will again be your general lifestyle.

- Herbs are only part of a natural food that you are taking in, you are adjusting the body in a very natural way, so diet must be part of that too.

The herbalist will advise you on your diet, how it may be lacking in calcium, for instance, or how it may be overdosing in chemical additives. Herbal supplements may be given in various forms, as tea, as oil to be massaged into certain parts of the body or put into a bath, or as a hand or foot soak to infuse through the skin. The type of combination of herbs is adjusted to the particular person's needs as is the concentration or dose. There are dozens of herbal tranquillisers,

115

sedatives and antidepressants, but these cannot be taken like their chemical equivalents. They are given to balance what the herbalist sees as 'deficiencies' or 'excesses' in the body and so have to be tailored to the individual's needs.

The herbalist we interviewed also recommended 'Bach flower remedies' for people with emotional problems. These can be obtained directly from a health shop.

Homoeopathy

Most practising homoeopaths have first trained as orthodox doctors. Homoeopathy is based on the idea that a symptom arises because the body's natural resistance mechanisms are working to repel an attack from germs, viruses, toxins or other invaders. So, rather than suppressing the symptom, we should help the resistance it is showing – on the principle of 'like cures like'.

A first visit to a homoeopath is much like going to an ordinary doctor except the case-history-taking is much longer and more detailed and the emphasis is on you as an individual rather than on the disease you may have.

Homoeopathic remedies are derived from herbs and minerals whose strength – or, more usually, dilution – are as important as the ingredients themselves. Although such remedies are available in health shops and chemists, it is unwise to take them unless you have first consulted a homoeopath.

Self-help groups

- Now I've been off the tablets for six months. It's been hard going and I could never have done it without the group really. We've met each other, we've made friends and we help each other get through. As we all get stronger, we can help those that are just coming off.

- It was a very great effort for me to go to Tranx the first time. I went almost a year ago. I didn't speak at all at those first few meetings. I went along and listened to everybody else and I thought I'm really not alone. And then I started to go regularly. There was a man there who had come off and he was wonderful and eventually with his encouragement and persuasion he got me to ride out the terrible withdrawal that I was going through.

Getting together with other people who share your problems can be supportive and there are now several self-help groups for people who are addicted to tranquillisers. Tranx, organised by Joan Jerome after she had spent 17 years on tranquillisers, has helped hundreds of people to come off pills and similar groups are being organised throughout Britain. Tranx has few resources and no trained therapists to teach relaxation or to counsel individual people. It operates mainly by mutual support. Much of this happens on the telephone, talking people through a panic attack or other crisis. There is also a small building where group meetings are held. A meeting usually involves people telling other members of the group about their experiences of tranquillisers and withdrawal.

At Tranx meetings, you can bring a partner or a friend so that they can understand what is happening to you and help support you. Often a partner finds it reassuring to realise there are others in the same situation.

Some other self-help groups arrange visits from therapists, who teach relaxation techniques or give talks on withdrawal problems.

There is a lot that you can do to help yourself in coming off tranquillisers and sleeping pills. Specific techniques like relaxation are included as part of the self-help withdrawal programme which follows.

9 Self-help withdrawal programme

Get ready

Coming off your tablets may not be easy. There will probably be times when you feel like giving up all your efforts and heading straight for the nearest supply. But remember, the more difficult it is for you to stop taking them, the more pleased you will be when you succeed. And if you can manage that, just think what else you could do!

There is no simple way of coming off. But we know that some ways are easier and better than others. This withdrawal programme will help you to cut down, and eventually to cut out your tablets altogether, in the way that best suits you. It will also show you how to cope without pills and how to deal with the temptation to go back on them.

Once you have decided to give the withdrawal programme a try, your first step should be to write down your reasons for making that decision. Looking back at these reasons will help you through the bad times later on. Here are some reasons that others have given for deciding to stop:

The pills are no longer helping me. I only continue to take them because I feel ill when I try to stop.

The problem for which I was prescribed these pills no longer exists. I don't need them any more.

I shall be able to think more clearly, have more energy and feel healthier.

I shall no longer be an addict.

My family will be proud of me.

I shall have greater self-respect.

Write down your reasons for deciding to come off

1

2

3

4

5

Tell someone in your family, or a friend, what you have decided to do. As well as providing support and encouragement, this person can help you in a practical way by keeping your tablets to make sure you don't cheat, taking your mind off your anxieties, helping with your daily chores and being available as much as possible. If you can talk to your doctor, it is also a good idea to tell him or her what you are planning to do.

During the GET READY phase of the withdrawal programme, get to know the kinds of symptom that you might experience while cutting down your tablets (see Chapter 7). If you do experience any of them, at least you will be prepared. You will know that you haven't developed a strange illness and that you are not going mad. However unpleasant, these symptoms are entirely due to the reduction of your tablets and will go away in time. Decide on a starting date. On that day, sign the contract below and then begin the GET STEADY phase, which lasts for two weeks. During this phase, put aside some time each day to learn how to cope without pills and how to resist temptation. You will then be ready to put this into practice when you reach GO.

From today I shall try my best to come off my tablets by keeping to the withdrawal programme

Signed........................... ....Date..................

Get steady

Before beginning to cut down your tablets, it is important to steady the dose you are taking at the moment. This means taking the same amount every day at fixed times of the day. By steadying your dose you will break the pattern of taking a tablet whenever you feel tense. If you are taking more than one type, tackle one at a time.

Take the same amount every day
People often take more tablets on some days than on others. You may take three on Monday if you have to cope with a very stressful event, forget to take your tablets altogether on Tuesday, take two on Wednesday because you don't feel very good, and so on. You must work out what is your *usual dose* and stick to that each day. This may not be the dose that your doctor has prescribed, but should be the dose that you take on average each day.

For example, Jane was prescribed 15mg of Valium a day by her doctor. She took this dose as one 5mg tablet three times a day. After a couple of years she began to take only two 5mg tablets a day. She has done so for several months now, which means that her *usual dose* is 10mg a day and not the 15mg that her doctor prescribed.

Veronica takes two 1mg tablets of Ativan on most days but occasionally has three 1mg tablets or only one 1mg tablet, according to how she feels. Her *usual dose* is 2mg Ativan a day.

If the number of tablets you take varies a lot from day to day, making it difficult to decide what is your *usual dose*, the following exercise will help you.

In the diary opposite write down the number of milligrams contained in each tablet you take. Do this before you take each tablet. If you leave it until afterwards it is very easy to forget. Every evening, add up the total number of milligrams you have taken on that day. Keep this diary for two weeks. By looking back at your diary after two weeks you will be able to work out your average daily dose. To do this, add together all your daily totals and then divide this number by 14. This figure is equivalent to your *usual dose*. If the answer doesn't

	day 1	day 2	day 3	day 4	day 5	day 6	day 7	day 8	day 9	day 10	day 11	day 12	day 13	day 14
Number of milligrams(mg) in first tablet														
Number of milligrams(mg) in second tablet														
Number of milligrams(mg) in third tablet														
Number of milligrams(mg) in fourth tablet														
Number of milligrams(mg) in fifth tablet														
Daily total														

come to a whole number, round it off by ignoring the fraction or decimal part.

Divide your daily dose into equal amounts

It is important at this stage to take your total dose for each day in *small amounts* rather than all at once. This will make it easier to cut down later. You should divide your daily dose into either three or four *equal portions*, depending on which is easier. You may have to break some tablets in half to do this.

If you take 10mg of Valium altogether on each day, for example, this divides best into five equal portions of 2mg. If you take 3mg of Ativan it is easy to divide this into three 1mg portions.

Whichever kind of tablet you take and whatever the dose, you must divide them each day into *small, equal* portions.

Take each portion of tablets at fixed times of the day

If your usual daily dose divides best into three equal portions, you have to decide on three times of the day when you are going to take your tablets. If you have four equal portions, decide on four times when you are going to take them. If you have three portions, you might decide to take one with breakfast, one with lunch and one with dinner at night. If you have four, you could have the last one at bedtime.

When deciding on the times of the day to take your tablets keep the following in mind:

(a) You must take your tablets at *exactly* the same times each day. It is no good deciding to have one at breakfast, one at lunch and one at dinner if you eat your meals at different times from day to day. Instead, you must decide on actual times of the day: 9.00 am, 1.00 pm and 7.00 pm, rather than mealtimes. If you skip lunch one day, or have dinner later than usual, you must still take your tablets at the fixed times. If your evening pill is due at 7.00 pm then you must always take it at 7.00 pm regardless of what you are doing at the time.

(b) The times of day that you take your tablets should be fairly evenly spaced. You might decide to take one in the morning, one in the afternoon, and one in the evening. You should not have finished all your tablets for the day by the middle of the afternoon.

(c) Before deciding at exactly what times you will take your tablets, ask yourself the following questions: 'At what time of day do I most need a tablet?' and 'At what time of day do I least need a tablet?'

Your answers will give you the two times of the day when you should take your tablets, one the most stressful time and the other the least stressful time. Decide on a time to take the remaining dose (or two doses if you have four portions of tablets a day) which falls between these two extremes. This might be a time of day when you sometimes take a tablet but not always, or a time of day when you take a tablet that you feel you could sometimes miss, or even a time of day when you feel you sometimes want to take a tablet but do not.

Rosalind, for example, has divided her tablets into three equal doses a day; one when she gets up at 7.00 am, one in the afternoon at 3.00 pm and one at 10.00 pm before she goes to bed. The most important tablet of the day for Rosalind is the one she takes in the morning with her tea before she gets out of bed. Without it she feels she couldn't face the day. This is when she feels most stressed. The time of day that she least wants a tablet is 10.00 pm. She has put her children to sleep, finished her tasks of the day, and is usually able to sit down and watch television for an hour or so before going to bed. This is when she feels most relaxed and never thinks of taking a tablet. A time when she usually takes a tablet is about 3.00 pm so that she feels able to cope with the children when they come home from school. Some days she feels she could do without this tablet and, occasionally, even forgets to take it. This is quite a stressful time of day for Rosalind. Much less so than first thing in the morning, but much more so than late evening.

Keep to this schedule for two weeks

It is important to take each of your tablet portions like clock-work for two weeks before beginning to cut down. You must take your pills at the fixed times, regardless of whether you need them or not at that particular moment. You must also stick to the same dose each time you take your pills, even when you feel anxious. Remember that you are taking the same amount as usual each day so the pills will have the same effect as before. Do not attempt to cut down your pills during these two weeks, even if you feel it would be easy to do so.

If you find it impossible to keep to this schedule, work out the maximum number of tablets you ever take in any one day and keep to this limit for two weeks.

Bottle up your pills

Put the exact amount of tablets that you will need for the two weeks in a bottle. If you need to break some in half to make the correct dose, you should do that now and not just before you are about to take them. You will then have the equal portions at your fingertips. It is a good idea to give these tablets, and any that you have left over, to a member of your family or a friend to keep so that you will avoid the temptation to increase your dose.

Keep a diary

To help you keep track of each tablet you take, you should keep a daily diary like the one opposite. This will help you in two ways: (a) To make sure you don't forget to take your tablets, or to check that you have already taken them, and (b) To decide which pills to cut down first when you begin to reduce.

Get steady daily diary

Keep this diary throughout the two weeks of the GET STEADY phase. *Before* you take each portion of tablet note the *time* and put a circle round the face which best describes how you feel. It is important to fill in the diary *each time* you take a tablet.

Week 1

Day		Time	very bad	bad	so-so	good	very good
1	1	am/pm	☹	☹	☺	☺	☺
	2	am/pm	☹	☹	☺	☺	☺
	3	am/pm	☹	☹	☺	☺	☺
	(4)	am/pm	☹	☹	☺	☺	☺
2	1	am/pm	☹	☹	☺	☺	☺
	2	am/pm	☹	☹	☺	☺	☺
	3	am/pm	☹	☹	☺	☺	☺
	(4)	am/pm	☹	☹	☺	☺	☺
3	1	am/pm	☹	☹	☺	☺	☺
	2	am/pm	☹	☹	☺	☺	☺
	3	am/pm	☹	☹	☺	☺	☺
	(4)	am/pm	☹	☹	☺	☺	☺
4	1	am/pm	☹	☹	☺	☺	☺
	2	am/pm	☹	☹	☺	☺	☺
	3	am/pm	☹	☹	☺	☺	☺
	(4)	am/pm	☹	☹	☺	☺	☺
5	1	am/pm	☹	☹	☺	☺	☺
	2	am/pm	☹	☹	☺	☺	☺
	3	am/pm	☹	☹	☺	☺	☺
	(4)	am/pm	☹	☹	☺	☺	☺
6	1	am/pm	☹	☹	☺	☺	☺
	2	am/pm	☹	☹	☺	☺	☺
	3	am/pm	☹	☹	☺	☺	☺
	(4)	am/pm	☹	☹	☺	☺	☺
7	1	am/pm	☹	☹	☺	☺	☺
	2	am/pm	☹	☹	☺	☺	☺
	3	am/pm	☹	☹	☺	☺	☺
	(4)	am/pm	☹	☹	☺	☺	☺

Week 2

Day   Time   Feelings

Day		Time	very bad	bad	so-so	good	very good
8	1	am/pm	☹	☹	☺	☺	☺
	2	am/pm	☹	☹	☺	☺	☺
	3	am/pm	☹	☹	☺	☺	☺
	(4)	am/pm	☹	☹	☺	☺	☺
9	1	am/pm	☹	☹	☺	☺	☺
	2	am/pm	☹	☹	☺	☺	☺
	3	am/pm	☹	☹	☺	☺	☺
	(4)	am/pm	☹	☹	☺	☺	☺
10	1	am/pm	☹	☹	☺	☺	☺
	2	am/pm	☹	☹	☺	☺	☺
	3	am/pm	☹	☹	☺	☺	☺
	(4)	am/pm	☹	☹	☺	☺	☺
11	1	am/pm	☹	☹	☺	☺	☺
	2	am/pm	☹	☹	☺	☺	☺
	3	am/pm	☹	☹	☺	☺	☺
	(4)	am/pm	☹	☹	☺	☺	☺
12	1	am/pm	☹	☹	☺	☺	☺
	2	am/pm	☹	☹	☺	☺	☺
	3	am/pm	☹	☹	☺	☺	☺
	(4)	am/pm	☹	☹	☺	☺	☺
13	1	am/pm	☹	☹	☺	☺	☺
	2	am/pm	☹	☹	☺	☺	☺
	3	am/pm	☹	☹	☺	☺	☺
	(4)	am/pm	☹	☹	☺	☺	☺
14	1	am/pm	☹	☹	☺	☺	☺
	2	am/pm	☹	☹	☺	☺	☺
	3	am/pm	☹	☹	☺	☺	☺
	(4)	am/pm	☹	☹	☺	☺	☺

Go

Prepare to cut down

Write down the order in which you are going to cut down your tablets. Begin with the one you could most easily do without, and end with the most difficult.

Looking back at your 'Get steady daily diary' will help you. It might be quite obvious that you feel worse before some tablets and not others. If you can find no clear pattern, write down the six times you felt *worst* and the six times you felt *best* before taking a tablet. Do your worst times tend to be at certain times of the day? What about your best times? This exercise should help you to order your tablets from the easiest to the most difficult to give up. If you are still not sure which tablets to cut down first, begin with the one you take latest in the day and work down to the one you take earliest.

If you take four portions of tablet a day, fill in List A.
If you take three portions of tablet a day, fill in List B.

List A
My *least* important tablet is at . . . . . . am/pm
My *second least* important tablet is at . . . . . . am/pm
My *second most* important tablet is at . . . . . . am/pm
My *most* important tablet is at . . . . . . am/pm

List B
My *least* important tablet is at . . . . . . am/pm
My *moderately* important tablet is at . . . . . . am/pm
My *most* important tablet is at . . . . . . am/pm

Cut down in stages

Cut down your tablets in stages, beginning with the portion that you need least and working up to the one that you need most. We shall discuss the time scheme in the next section. If you are taking three portions a day, cut down your tablets in six stages; if you are taking four, cut down in eight stages.

Eight stages will not necessarily take longer than six to complete because less time might be spent at each.

Stage 1
Cut out half of your *least* important tablet

Stage 2
Cut out the other half

Stage 3
Cut out half of your *second least* important tablet

Stage 4
Cut out the other half

Stage 5
Cut out half of your *second most* important tablet

Stage 6
Cut out the other half

Stage 7
Cut out half of your *most* important tablet

Stage 8
Cut out the other half

If you find it impossible to cut down in this way, set yourself a maximum limit of tablets that you will take each day and keep to this limit until you feel ready to reduce to a lower limit.

Cut down at your own pace
The more gradually you reduce your tablets, the less likely you are to have withdrawal symptoms and the less severe they are likely to be. But this does not necessarily mean that it is best to withdraw slowly. You might feel that you want to come off your tablets quickly – even if you suffer from bad withdrawal symptoms – so as not to prolong the agony.

As withdrawal symptoms can take some time to develop after you reduce your dose, you should remain at each stage for at least one week before moving on to the next stage. This means that the minimum time you will take to come off your tablets is six weeks if you begin by taking three portions a day, and eight weeks if you begin with four portions a day. It is very likely that you will need to remain at some stages for several weeks before you feel ready to move on to the next one, particularly as you near the end. It is not unusual to take several months to come off the tablets altogether, and some people need a year or more.

Until you begin to reduce your tablets you will not know how you are going to feel. Everyone reacts differently and there is no way of knowing exactly what symptoms, if any, you will experience, when you will have them, or how long they will last. Do not move from one stage to the next unless your withdrawal symptoms have disappeared or are at a bearable level. It is better to take a little longer to come off than to reduce so quickly that you are unable to cope and find yourself back at square one.

It is not just withdrawal symptoms which make it difficult to cut down. Any habit is hard to break, and taking pills can become a habit like any other. If you are used to taking a tablet whenever you feel anxious, it can be difficult to break that pattern, even when you do not have bad withdrawal symptoms. Pills mask the normal anxiety which we all feel when we are under stress. So cutting down slowly will give you more time to get used to dealing with these feelings again and to learn to cope in other ways with life's problems.

Recording your progress
Whenever you take a portion of tablets, write the *time* and the *dose* in a notebook, which you should keep specially for this purpose. This record will enable you to keep track of your progress.

Date	Time	Dose
	8am	5mg
	1pm	2.5mg
	8pm	5mg
Total daily dose		12.5mg
	8am	5mg
	8pm	5mg
Total daily dose		10mg

You can also keep a visual record of your progress by putting a cross on the graph below at the end of each week.

Look at the column on the graph which corresponds to the week of the withdrawal programme which you have just finished. Run a finger up the vertical column until you come to the number which corresponds to the stage you have reached. Put a cross at this point. Join up the crosses for each week as you go along by drawing a straight line between them. After 18 weeks, draw another graph and keep going.

Stage

8

7

6

5

4

3

2

1

  1 2 3 4 5 6 7 8 9 10 11 12 13 14 15 16 17 18
                                                        Week

Reward yourself

Reward yourself every time you move from one stage to the next. You deserve it!

An important reward is, of course, the satisfaction of knowing that you have done well. Put all the tablets you cut out in a bottle so that you can see just how many you have managed not to take. Make sure you actually tell yourself how pleased you are, and remind yourself of the benefits of coming off. This will help you to continue to be successful.

You could also give yourself a treat or a present. Before you begin to cut down, make a list of the rewards you will give yourself after completing each stage:

1

2

3

4

5

6

Coping while you come off

These methods are for you to use when you feel bad. You will also be able to use them after you come off.

Relaxation

Relaxation is a useful technique whenever you feel anxious. It will teach you how to tell when you are becoming tense, and how to relax instead. Learning to relax is like any new skill – it takes practice. You may find relaxation difficult at first but it will soon become easier. It is very like learning to swim or to ride a bicycle. Your body has to learn to respond in a new way.

Practice relaxation twice a day or more for at least 15 minutes each time.

Preparation

Sit in a comfortable chair or, better still, lie down. Choose a quiet, warm room where you will not be interrupted. Take off your shoes and loosen any tight clothing.

If you are sitting, uncross your legs and rest your arms along the arms of the chair.

If you are lying down, lie on your back with your legs uncrossed and your arms by your side.

Close your eyes and be aware of your body. Notice how you are breathing and identify the muscles which feel tense. Make sure you are comfortable.

Breathing

Start to breathe slowly and deeply. Expand your abdomen as you breathe IN and then raise your rib cage to let more air in until your lungs are filled right to the top. Hold your breath for a couple of seconds. Then slowly breathe OUT, allowing your rib cage and stomach to relax, and your lungs to empty completely. Do not strain. With practice it will become much easier. After your breathing pattern is established, start the muscle relaxation exercises.

Keep this slow, rhythmic breathing going throughout the relaxation session. Remember to keep your eyes closed all the time.

Muscle relaxation

Muscle relaxation is learned by alternately tensing and relaxing different muscle groups. This will teach you the difference between the physical sensations of tension and relaxation, and will help you to reduce muscle tension.

Go through each of the 10 muscle groups below, one at a time. TENSE the muscles for five seconds and then RELAX them for 20 seconds. If you feel that a muscle group is still tense, you may repeat it for a second time, or even a third time, before going on to the next group.

To relax each muscle group effectively you need to talk yourself through both the tension and the relaxation phases. Here are some instructions which you should say SILENTLY to yourself as you go through each muscle group. You will soon learn the muscle relaxation instructions by heart.

Begin with your feet:

Tense up
Tense your muscles slightly – don't strain them
Hold it
Feel the tension in your muscles
Notice where the tightness is
Keep your muscles tense
Concentrate on the tension
Relax
Feel the tension leave your muscles
Feel them grow more and more relaxed
Feel them become heavier and heavier
Feel the warmth flow through them
Feel the tension drain away
Notice the difference between tension and relaxation
Let all the tension go
Feel warm and heavy
Say words like 'calm' and 'relax' silently to yourself
Feel more and more relaxed
Let this feeling increase

Go through each muscle group in order:
1 Curl your toes and press your feet down
2 Now tense your calf muscles
3 Now tense your thighs, straighten your knees and make your legs stiff
4 Now make your buttocks tight
5 Now tense your stomach
6 Now clench your fists
7 Now bend your elbows and tense your arms
8 Now hunch your shoulders
9 Now press your head back into a cushion to tense your neck muscles
10 Now clench your jaws, frown and screw up your eyes

Relaxing thoughts

Once you have completed the sequence from 1 to 10, keep your eyes closed and keep breathing slowly and deeply. Let your whole body become more and more deeply relaxed for a few minutes longer without first tensing your muscles. Be aware of the feelings of heaviness and physical well-being spreading through your body.

To become deeply relaxed you must not only work on your muscles but also relax your mind. If you are worrying about work, shopping for the evening meal, or anything at all, you will not be able to relax properly. While you continue to relax, imagine a pleasant scene, any scene at all that you find relaxing. Try to 'see' it as clearly as you can in your mind's eye, concentrating on it for several minutes. For example, you might imagine taking a walk along the shore of a deserted beach, surrounded by mountains, in the middle of summer. Really feel that you are right inside that scene. Hear the water lapping against the shore and the sound of the seagulls, smell the sea air, feel the sun on your skin. Think about what you can see. Feel as if you are really there. Or, you might imagine sitting in front of a log fire in winter feeling very snug and warm. Hear the fire crackling and the rain beating against the window pane, see the flames leap up the chimney, feel the heat of the fire and smell the woody smoke.

Spend a few minutes imagining your pleasant scene. Don't forget to continue to breathe slowly and deeply and to keep your eyes closed.

Ending the session

Just before you end the relaxation session, say the word 'relax' silently to yourself a few times when you breathe out. This will help you to associate the word with the feeling. Then silently tell yourself that when you open your eyes you will be perfectly relaxed but alert. Count silently to three and open your eyes.

Points to remember

Concentrate on your breathing and the instructions you give yourself. Don't let distracting thoughts enter your mind – they will prevent you from becoming fully relaxed.

Don't strain your muscles – just make them tense enough to feel the difference between tension and relaxation.

Don't worry if you become a bit dizzy, or notice tingling sensations, or feel your muscles jerk. These are all signs of relaxation and are not uncommon. If this happens try to breathe less heavily.

Quick relaxation

Once you have mastered deep relaxation it is useful to learn how to speed up this process to help you cope with stress anywhere and at any time during the day. After all, we can't lie down in a supermarket or at the office for a 20-minute session. Relaxing more quickly may be difficult at first, but will soon become easier. Begin by practising step 1 a few times each day. Move on to step 2 only when you feel ready to do so, and then to step 3, and so on. Make sure that you are happy with each step before moving on to the next.

Step 1

Instead of tensing and relaxing one group of muscles at a time, do this with several at once. Group the following muscles:
(a) feet and legs
(b) buttocks and stomach
(c) hands, arms and shoulders
(d) neck and face
First close your eyes and begin to breathe slowly and deeply. Then go through each of these four groups, tensing and relaxing all the muscles in each group in the same way as you did for each of the 10 muscle groups. After relaxing your muscles, spend a few minutes thinking relaxing thoughts and end the session in the usual way by first saying 'relax' silently to yourself a few times when you breathe out.

Step 2

Once you are able to relax deeply using the four muscle groups, go through the same procedure with only two muscle groups:

(a) lower body – feet, legs, buttocks and stomach

(b) upper body – hands, arms, shoulders, neck and face

Step 3

Relax your whole body at once by tensing all the muscles together to make your body stiff as you breathe in, and then relax. Don't forget to think relaxing thoughts for a few minutes before ending the session in the usual way.

Step 4

You have been tensing your muscles before relaxing them so that you could learn to identify tension in your body and become aware of the difference between tension and relaxation. By now you should know how your muscles feel when they are tense and be able to recognise which ones need to relax.

No longer tense your muscles before relaxing. Instead, sit or lie down and simply think about which parts of your body are tense before relaxing in the usual way. Remember to keep your eyes closed and to breathe slowly and deeply. Spend a few minutes thinking of a pleasant scene and say the word 'relax' silently to yourself a few times before you end the session.

Step 5

Your final goal is to be able to relax whenever you begin to feel tense, wherever you happen to be at the time.

Make yourself as comfortable as possible
Begin to breathe slowly and deeply
Focus your attention on the tension
Relax your muscles
Say RELAX silently each time you breathe out

Practise several times each day. It is a good idea to get into the habit of relaxing for a few seconds whenever you do certain routine activities, whether or not you feel tense – perhaps when you are about to have a cup of tea, or speak on the telephone. This will help prevent tension from building up.

Using your imagination
You can use your imagination to conjure up in your mind situations which make you feel anxious. If you do this while you are deeply relaxed you can practise dealing with the unpleasant feelings of anxiety when you are not actually being threatened. This will give you practice in using relaxation to reduce the anxiety produced by stressful situations thus helping you to cope with them when they occur in real life.
A word of caution – Although many people find this technique very helpful it does not work for everyone, and some people find that it makes them even more anxious.

Preparation
Think of a specific activity which makes you feel anxious. This might be travelling on a bus or going to a supermarket. Then make a list of up to 10 situations which are associated with this activity. The list should include situations which make you feel just a little anxious, like thinking about travelling on a bus or standing at a bus stop, right up to those which make you feel very anxious indeed and which you may avoid altogether, like sitting on the top deck of a crowded bus.

1

2

3

4

5

6

7

8

9

10

Put the activities in order from the least to the most stressful situation.

1

2

3

4

5

6

7

8

9

10

The exercise
This exercise should be done towards the end of a relaxation session when you are feeling deeply relaxed.
1   Imagine yourself to be in the situation at the top of your list for about 30 seconds – the one which makes you feel least anxious. Really feel as if you are there.
2   If you feel anxious STOP imagining this situation. Instead, switch your attention to relaxing as deeply as you can, saying the word RELAX silently to yourself each time you breathe out.

3   When you begin to feel relaxed, concentrate on the pleasant scene which you use during relaxation.

4   Repeat this procedure of imagining the stressful situation, and then relaxing, two or three times in each session.

5   When you are sure your first situation does not make you feel anxious, move on to the next, and so on.

At first you will probably have difficulty in relaxing as deeply as usual because you have been imagining a stressful situation. This will become much easier with practice.

From imagination to reality

Once you are able to imagine a stressful situation without becoming anxious, the next stage is to try to cope with that situation in real life. Only by trying will you be able to discover that it may not be as bad as you feared.

Do this gradually. For example, if sitting on a bus makes you anxious, start with an uncrowded bus on a Sunday afternoon, then gradually progress, step-by-step, to taking the bus during a weekday rush hour. When you are in the bus relax as much as you can. You will probably become more and more anxious at first but this feeling will reach a peak and then diminish after a few minutes. *It is important to stay in the situation until the initial increase in anxiety goes down and you feel more comfortable.* Use relaxation to overcome it. Saying to yourself statements like 'I can do it', 'stay here just a little longer' and 'this feeling will soon disappear' will also help. Stay on the bus for long enough to allow your anxiety to subside. Taking a friend with you can provide the support and encouragement you need to persevere.

If you do not manage to stay in the situation, try again as soon as possible. If you are unsuccessful a second time, then try to make the situation a little easier.

Return to the stressful situation every day and try to remain there for a little longer each time until it no longer makes you feel anxious. Then begin this procedure again with a more stressful situation, and so on.

Step-by-step
If you find that you can't cope with something that is looming ahead, do it step-by-step. Concentrate on one step at a time, then stop and switch to something you enjoy before returning to the next step. A good way of dividing up a task is to decide to stop after a fixed period of time, whether you have finished or not, and then do something pleasant. You can even use this technique to plan your day. Write down all the tasks that you have to do along with the times when you are going to do them. Put a time limit on the ones you don't enjoy and try to include as many pleasant activities as possible.

When you are faced with a problem, tackle that step-by-step, too.

1 Make sure you are absolutely clear about what the problem is. Be as specific as possible.
2 Think of as many different solutions to the problem as you can.
3 Decide on which solution seems best.
4 Try out that solution to see how well it works. If it is not effective, try another.

Resisting temptation

There will no doubt be times during the withdrawal programme when you feel like giving it all up. Here are some ways to help you resist temptation:

The temptation test
As soon as you feel tempted to take an extra pill, write down in your notebook:

> The time
> Where you are
> What you are doing
> Who you are with
> How you feel

Then draw a scale like the one shown here.

Desperate to have a pill

|

No desire to have a pill

Put a mark on it according to how you feel *at that moment*.

Desperate to have a pill

|

No desire to have a pill

Now try to resist temptation by using one of these methods:
change the way you think (p. 143), **talk to yourself** (p. 144) *or*
do something different (p. 145)
Immediately afterwards, go back and mark the scale, according to how you feel *now*.

Desperate to have a pill

╳ Before

╳ After

No desire to have a pill

Also note down which method you used to *resist temptation*.
Do this exercise whenever you feel tempted.

Here are two examples:

Desperate to have a pill

	Time: 2.30pm
✗ Before	Where: At the office
	What: Made to work late
After	Who: Supervisor
	How: Tense. Worried I am late
	for children
No desire to have a pill	METHOD: Talk to myself

Desperate to have a pill

✗ Before	Time: 4pm
	Where: At home
✗ After	What: Housework
	Who: Alone
	How: Panicky. Afraid I shall faint
No desire to have a pill	METHOD: Relaxation

You may find that at first there is little difference in how you feel before and after the exercise. But with practice you will soon be able to keep temptation at bay. Your notes will show you which ways of RESISTING TEMPTATION work best for you.

Look back at your notebook to pinpoint the circumstances which make you most tempted to take a tablet. Use the methods you have learned for COPING WITHOUT PILLS to prepare yourself the next time they crop up. You may not be able to get rid of feelings of temptation altogether. The main thing is to keep them under control.

Once you are able to reduce your desire to take a tablet, try lasting a little longer each time before using one of the techniques to help you resist. As soon as you feel tempted, mark the scale as usual and then *time yourself* to see how long you can last. You will find that you can put up with these feelings of temptation for longer than you think without giving in to them.

Change the way you think

If you focus your attention on the thoughts going through your mind whenever you feel tempted to give up the withdrawal programme, you will probably find that you are looking at things in a particularly negative way. Changing the way you think will help you cope with feeling bad and help you to persevere. To do this you must first recognise your negative thoughts and then challenge them by substituting more realistic ones. Look at the following examples:

Negative thoughts	*Realistic thoughts*
I am a failure.	I have already managed to cut out one tablet. I have done well.
If I don't have a pill I shan't be able to clean the house.	It doesn't matter. It is more important to keep to the withdrawal programme.
I can't bear these feelings.	I have managed so far. I can try a little longer.
If I don't have a pill I shall go crazy.	I won't go crazy. I may feel bad for a while but it won't last for ever.
I never succeed at anything.	I have done lots of good things. I am only thinking this way because I feel bad right now.
I don't feel well enough to cook the dinner.	So what! Perhaps I could ask my husband to help me until I feel better.

I can't go through with it.	I can go through with it but I know I shall feel bad for a while.
I have so much to do.	I don't have to do it all today. I am going to put myself first until I feel better.
This is a bad time for me to give up. I have too many worries at the moment.	I always have worries. Now is as good a time as any.
My husband is getting fed up with me feeling this way.	I haven't actually discussed it with him. I don't know what he feels.
I felt so bad yesterday I couldn't go out.	But I did do other things at home.

As soon as you begin to think about giving up the withdrawal programme write down all the negative thoughts that go through your mind.

Then write down other more realistic ways of thinking about how you feel.

Talk to yourself
Feelings of temptation can be influenced by the things you say to yourself. So talking to yourself can help you overcome the urge to take an extra tablet; saying *out loud* statements such as:

Stop

Think before you swallow

This feeling won't last

I can control it

Don't give up now

I have done well to get this far – don't spoil it now

Has all my effort been for nothing?

How shall I feel about this in an hour from now?

These are examples of statements which are effective for others. Those which will help *you* may be different.

Write down 10 statements that you might actually say to yourself if you wanted to stop yourself from taking an extra pill.

Thinking about the self-defeating thoughts which go through your head when you want to take an extra tablet will help you to do this.

1

2

3

4

5

6

7

8

9

10

Write each statement on a separate card and keep them with you at all times. Whenever you are tempted to give up the withdrawal programme, read each card *out loud* and *as if you really mean it.*

Do something different
Take your mind off the urge to swallow a tablet by doing something active. Here are some suggestions:

Make a cup of tea

Phone a friend

Count backwards from 100 to 1
Read a magazine
Knit or sew
Sing or dance to music
Take a walk
Do some gardening
Go for a run
Have a bath

You may find it difficult to distract yourself at first but with practice it will become much easier. Try to concentrate on what you are doing rather than on what you feel.

Giving in to temptation

Having 'just one' extra pill does not mean that all is lost, but it does mean that you are more likely to give in altogether.

If you do lapse, make sure this doesn't turn into a total relapse. Don't make excuses such as:

I am a failure
Once an addict, always an addict
I just can't manage without pills
I don't have the willpower

If these statements were true you wouldn't have managed to get this far! You will feel much better if you can say, 'Well done. Even though I had one extra pill, I went straight back on the withdrawal programme', instead of, 'It's no good. Now I have had an extra pill I may as well give up altogether.'

Use the lapse as a way of learning how not to give in again. Do not blame yourself. Just think carefully about the circumstances which led up to the lapse so that you will be better prepared next time. You have not failed – it just might take a bit longer than you think to come off.

If ever you do have 'just one' extra pill write down the advantages and disadvantages of lapsing and give each a score like this:

5 – very large gain or loss
4 – large gain or loss
3 – moderate gain or loss
2 – small gain or loss
1 – very small gain or loss

For example:

Advantages	*Gain* (1–5)	*Disadvantages*	*Loss* (1–5)
I felt more relaxed	3	I felt guilty	5
I could go shopping	2	Pill less effective than expected	3
TOTAL =	5	TOTAL =	8

Now look back at the list of reasons for deciding to come off which you made during the GET READY *phase. Try to think of more disadvantages of having just one pill. Do the disadvantages outweigh the advantages?*

You may find that you begin to lapse once you reach a certain stage of the withdrawal programme – perhaps when you are down to your last tablet. Maybe you have moved to the next stage before you are ready? In this case it is often a good idea to remain at the previous one for a bit longer. But don't stay there for too long or you will never manage to come off at all. The last stage or two are often the most difficult, but once you have overcome these, you will have reached your goal!

GOOD LUCK!

References

Chapter 1

1 Lader, M. (1981) 'Epidemic in the making: benzodiazepine dependence', *Epidemiological Impact of Psychotropic Drugs* (Tognoni, Bellantuono and Lader, eds.). Elsevier/North Holland Biomedical Press.

2 Petursson, H. and Lader, M. (1981) 'Benzodiazepine Dependence', *British Journal of Addiction,* **76**, 133–45.

3 Cooperstock, R. (1976) 'Psychotropic drug use among women', *Canadian Medical Association Journal*, **115**, 760–3.
Mellinger, G. D. and Balter, M. B. (1981) 'Prevalence and patterns of use of psychotherapeutic drugs: results from a 1979 survey of American adults', *Epidemiological Impact*, op. cit.
Skegg, D. C. G., Doll, R. and Perry, J. (1977) 'Use of medicines in general practice', *British Medical Journal*, **1**, 1561–5.

4 *Australian Health Survey 1977–8*, Catalogue No. 4311 (1979). Australian Bureau of Statistics, Canberra.
Balter, M. B., Levine, J . and Mannheimer, D. I. (1974). 'Cross-national study of the extent of anti-anxiety/sedative drug use', *New England Journal of Medicine*, **290,** 769–784.
Cooperstock, R. and Parnell, P. (1980) 'Prevalence and patterns of use of psychotropic substances', *Expert Committee on the Implementation of the Convention of Psychotropic Substances*. World Health Organisation, Geneva, 15–20 September.
Jones, I., Simpson, D., Brown, A. C., Bainton, D. and McDonald, H. (1984) 'Prescribing psychotropic drugs in general practice: three year study', *British Medical Journal*, **289**, 1045–8, 20 October.
Khan, A., Hornblow, A. R. and Walshe, J. W. B. (1981) 'Benzo-

diazepine dependence: a general practice survey', *New Zealand Medical Journal*, **94**, 19–21.

5 Penfold, P. S. and Walker, G. A. (1983) *Women and the Psychiatric Paradox*. Eden Press, London.

6 *A Socio-Demographic Profile of People Prescribed Mood-Modifiers*, Final Report, January. (1978) Research Division, Saskatchewan Alcoholism Commission.

7 Ehrenreich, B. and English, D. (1976) *Complaints and Disorders: The Sexual Politics of Sickness*. Writers and Readers, London.

Chapter 3

1 Tyrer, P. (1980) 'Dependence on benzodiazepines', *British Journal of Psychiatry*, **137**, 576–7.

2 Williams, P., Murray, J. and Clare, A. (1982) 'A longitudinal study of psychotropic drug prescription', *Psychological Medicine*, **12**, 201–7.

3 Gove, W. R., Hughes, M. and Style, C. B. (1983) 'Does marriage have positive effects on the psychological well-being of the individual?' *Journal of Health and Social Behaviour*, **24**, 122–31.
Williams, J. (1984) 'Women and Mental Illness', *Psychology Survey* (Nicholson and Beloff, eds.) British Psychological Society.

4 Marks, J. N., Goldberg, D. P. and Hillier, V. F. (1979) 'Determinants of the ability of general practitioners to detect psychiatric illness', *Psychological Medicine*, **9**, 337–53.

5 Gove, W. R. (1981) 'Sex differences in the epidemiology of mental disorder: evidence and explanations', *Gender and Disordered Behaviour: Sex Differences in Psychopathology* (Gomberg and Franks, eds.). Brunner/Mazel, New York.

6 Guse, L., Morier, G. and Ludwig, J. (October 1976) 'Winnipeg Survey of Prescription (Mood-Altering) use among Women', *Technical Report*. NMUDD Manitoba Alcoholism Foundation.

7 Briscoe, M. (1982) 'Sex differences in psychological well-being', *Psychological Medicine*, Monograph Supplement 1.
Mostow, E. and Newberry, P. (1975) 'Work role and depression

in women: a comparison of workers and housewives in treatment', *American Journal of Orthopsychiatry*, **45**, 538–48.

8 Cafferata, G. L., Kaspar, J. and Bernstein, A. (1983) 'Family roles, structure and stressors in relation to sex differences in obtaining psychotropic drugs', *Journal of Health and Social Behaviour*, **24**, 132–43.

9 Mellinger and Balter, 'Prevalence and patterns of use of psychotherapeutic drugs', *Epidemiological Impact*, op. cit.

10 Murray, J., Dunn, G., Williams, P. and Tanopolsky, A. (1981) 'Factors affecting the consumption of psychotropic drugs', *Psychological Medicine*, **11**, 551–60.

11 Parry, H. J., Balter, M. B., Mellinger, G. D., Cisin, I. H. and Manheimer, D. I. (1973) 'National patterns of psychotherapeutic drug use', *Archives of General Psychiatry*, **28**, 769–83.

12 Cooperstock, R. (1971) 'Sex differences in the use of mood-modifying drugs', *Journal of Health and Social Behaviour*, **12**, 238–44.

13 Williams, P., Murray, J. and Clare, A. (1982) 'A longitudinal study of psychotropic drug prescription', *Psychological Medicine*, **12**, 201–6.

Chapter 4

1 Brown, G. W. and Harris, T. (1978) *Social Origins of Depression: A Study of Psychiatric Disorder in Women*. Tavistock, London.

2 Nairne, K. and Smith, G. (1984) *Dealing with Depression*. Women's Press, London.

3 Cleary, P. D. and Mechanic, D. (1982) 'Sex differences in psychological well-being', *Psychiatric Medicine*, Monograph Supplement 1.

4 Krause, N. (1984) 'Employment outside the home and the woman's psychological well-being', *Social Psychiatry*, **19**, 41–8.
Warr, P. and Parry, G. (1982) 'Depressed mood in working-class mothers with and without paid employment', *Social Psychiatry*, **17**, 161–5.
Warr, P. and Parry, G. (1982) 'Paid employment and women's

psychological well-being', *Psychological Bulletin*, **91**, 498–516.

5 Shaver, P. and Freedman, J. (1976) 'Your pursuit of happiness', *Psychology Today*, **10**, 26–32.

6 Briscoe, M. (1982) 'Sex differences in psychological well-being', *Psychological Medicine*, Monograph Supplement 1.

7 Ibid.

8 Cleary, P. D. and Mechanic, D. (1983). 'Sex differences in psychological distress among married people', *Journal of Health and Social Behaviour*, **24**, 111–21.
Moss, P. and Plavis, I. (1977) Mental Distress in Mothers of Pre-school Children in Inner London. *Psychological Medicine*, **7**, 641–52.
Richman, N. (1976) 'Depression in Mothers of Pre-school Children', *Journal of Child Psychology and Psychiatry*, **17**, 75–8.

9 Brown and Harris. *Social Origins of Depression*, op. cit.

10 Cleary and Mechanic. 'Sex differences in psychological distress', *Journal of Health*, op. cit.

11 Oakley, A. (1982) *Subject Women*. Fontana, London.

12 Murray Parkes, C. (1975). *Bereavement: Studies of Grief in Adult Life*. Penguin, Harmondsworth.

13 Brown and Harris. *Social Origins of Depression*, op. cit. Henderson, S., Duncan-Jones, P., McAuley, H. and Ritchie, K. (1979) 'The Patient's Primary Group', *Psychosocial Disorders in General Practice* (Williams and Clare, eds.). Academic Press, New York.

14 Briscoe. 'Sex differences in psychological well-being', op. cit.

15 Kessler, R. C., Brown, R. L. and Broman, C. L. (1981) 'Sex differences in psychiatric help-seeking: Evidence from four large-scale surveys', *Journal of Health and Social Behaviour*, **22**, 49–64.

Chapter 5

1 Cooperstock, R. (1971) 'Sex differences in the use of mood-modifying drugs', *Journal of Health and Social Behaviour*, **12**, 238–44.

Cooperstock, R. (1976) 'Psychotropic drug use among women', *Canadian Medical Association Journal*, **115**, 760–3.

Cooperstock, R. and Parnell, P. (1980) 'Prevalence and patterns of use of psychotropic substances', *Expert Committee on the Implementation of the Convention of Psychotropic Substances*. World Health Organisation, Geneva, 15–20 September.

Jones, I., Simpson, D., Brown, A. C., Baintaon, D. and McDonald, H. (1984) 'Prescribing psychotropic drugs in general practice: three-year study', *British Medical Journal*, **289**, 1045–8, 20 October.

Mellinger, G. D., Balter, M. B. and Manheimer, D. I. (1971) 'Patterns of psychotherapeutic drug use among adults in San Francisco', *Archives of General Psychiatry*, **25**, 385–94.

Murray, J., Dunn, G., Williams, P. and Tarnopolsky, A. (1981) Factors affecting the consumption of psychotropic drugs. *Psychological Medicine*, **11**, 551–60.

2 Marks, J. N., Goldberg, D. P. and Hillier, V. F. (1979) 'Determinants of the ability of general practitioners to detect psychiatric illness', *Psychological Medicine*, **9**, 337–53.

3 Byrne, P. S. and Long, P. E. (1976) *Doctors Talking to Patients*. HMSO, London.

4 Roberts, H. (1985) *Patient Patients*. Pandora Press, London.

5 Chambers, C. D., White, O. Z. and Lindquist, H. L. (1983) 'Physician attitudes and prescribing practices: a focus on minor tranquillizers', *Journal of Psychoactive Drugs*, **15**, 55–9.

6 Marks et al. 'Determinants', op. cit.

7 Savage, R. and Wilson, A. (1977) 'Doctors' attitudes to women in medicine', *Journal of the Royal College of General Practitioners*, **27**, 363–5.

8 Chambers et al. 'Physician attitudes', op. cit.

9 Hull, F. M. and Hull, F. S. (1984) 'Time and the general practitioner: the patient's view', *Journal of the Royal College of General Practitioners*, **37**, 71–5.

10 Wheatley, D. (1979) 'Evaluation of psychotropic drugs in general practice', *Psychosocial Disorders in General Practice* (Williams and Clare, eds.). Academic Press, New York.

11 Parish, P. A. (1971) 'The prescribing of psychotropic drugs in

general practice', *Journal of the Royal College of General Practitioners*, Supplement 4, **21**, 1–77.

12 Stimpson, G. (1975) 'Women in a doctored world', *New Society*, 265–7. May.

13 Cooperstock, R. (1979) 'Some factors involved in the increased prescribing of psychotropic drugs', *Psychosocial Disorders in General Practice* (Williams and Clare, eds.). Academic Press, New York.

14 Quoted by R. Cooperstock, op. cit., p. 169.

15 Stimpson, 'Women in a doctored world', op. cit.

16 Griffiths, D. (1981) 'Psychological aspects of the response to drugs', *Psychology and Medicine* (Griffiths, ed.). Macmillan, London.

Chapter 6

1 Lader, M. and Marks, I. M. (1971) *Clinical Anxiety*. Heinemann Medical, London.

2 Noyes, R., Clancy, J., Hoenk, P. R. and Slyman, D. J. (1980) 'The prognosis of anxiety neurosis', *Archives of General Psychiatry*, **37**, 173–8.

3 Marks, I. M. (1969). *Fears and Phobias*. Heinemann Medical, London.

4 Mathews, A. M., Gelder, M. G. and Johnston, D. W. (1981) *Agoraphobia: Nature and Treatment*. Guilford Press, New York.

5 Hamilton, M. (1982) 'Symptoms and assessment of depression', *Handbook of Affective Disorders* (Paykel, ed.). Churchill Livingstone, London and New York.

6 Oswald, I. (1984) 'Insomnia', *British Journal of Hospital Medicine*, 219–24, March.

7 Murray, R. M. and McGuffin, P. (1983) 'Genetic aspects of mental disorders', *Companion to psychiatric studies* (Kendall and Zeally, eds.). Churchill Livingstone, London and New York.

8 Rutter, M. and Madge, N. (1976) *Cycles of Disadvantage*. Heinemann, London.

9 Paykel, E. S. (1978) 'Contribution of life-events to causation of psychiatric illness', *Psychological Medicine*, **8**, 245–53.

10 Finlay-Jones, R. A. and Brown, G. W. (1981) 'Types of stressful life-event and the onset of anxiety and depressive disorders', *Psychological Medicine*, **11**, 803–15.

11 Abramson, L. Y., Seligman, M. E. P. and Teasdale, J. D. (1978) 'Learned helplessness in humans: critique and reformulation', *Journal of Abnormal Psychology*, **87**, 49–74.

12 Kendall, R. E. (1983) 'Affective Psychoses', *Companion to Psychiatric Studies*, op. cit.

13 Clare, A. W. (1979) 'Psychiatric and social aspects of premenstrual complaints in women attending general practitioners', *Emotion and Reproduction* (Carenza and Zichella, eds.). Academic Press, London.

14 Osborn, M. (1984) 'Depression at the menopause', *British Journal of Hospital Medicine*, 126–9, September.

15 Snaith, P. R. (1983) 'Pregnancy-related psychiatric disorder', *British Journal of Hospital Medicine*, 450–6, May.

16 Henderson, A. S. (1984) 'Interpreting the evidence on social support', *Social Psychiatry*, **19**, 49–52.

Chapter 7

1 Rickels, K. (1980) *Benzodiazepines: Use and misuse*. Paper presented to the Annual Meeting of the American Psychopathological Association, Washington DC, March.

2 Committee on the Review of Medicines. (1980) 'Systematic review of the benzodiazepines', *British Medical Journal*, 910–12, 29 March.

3 Lader, M. and Petursson, H. (1983). 'Rational use of anxiolytic/sedative drugs', *Drugs*, **25**, 514–28.

4 Goldberg, H. and DiMascio, A. (1978) 'Psychotropic drugs in pregnancy', *Psychopharmacology: A generation of progress* (Lipton, DiMascio and Killam, eds.). Raven Press, New York.

5 Owen, R. T. and Tyrer, P. (1983) Benzodiazepine dependence: A review of the evidence. *Drugs*, **25**, 385–98.

6 Schopf, J. (1983) 'Withdrawal phenomena after long-term administration of benzodiazepines: A review of recent investigations', *Pharmacopsychiatry*, **16**, 1–8.

7 Marks, J. (1978) *The benzodiazepines. Use, Overuse, Misuse, Abuse*. MTP Press, Lancaster.

8 Lader, M. (1983) 'Dependence on benzodiazepines', *Journal of Clinical Psychiatry*, **44**, 121–7.

9 Ashton, H. (1984) 'Benzodiazepine withdrawal: An unfinished story', *British Medical Journal*, 1135–40, 14 April.

10 Hollister, L. (1981) 'Current antidepressant drugs: Their clinical use', *Drugs*, **22**, 129–52.

11 Blackwell, B. (1981) 'Adverse effects of antidepressant drugs. Part 1: Monoamine Oxidase Inhibitors and Tricyclics', *Drugs*, **21**, 201–19.

12 Ibid. 'Part 2: Second generation antidepressants and rational decision making in antidepressant therapy', 273–82.

Chapter 8

1 Fonagy, P. and Higgitt, A. (1984) *Personality theory and clinical practice*. Methuen, London and New York.

2 Robson, M. H., France, R. and Bland, M. (1984) 'Clinical psychologists in primary care: Controlled clinical and economic evaluation', *British Medical Journal*, **288**, 1805–8, 16 June.

3 Rosen, G. M. (1977) *The Relaxation Book*. Prentice-Hall, New Jersey.

4 Bellack, A. S. and Hersen, M. (1977) *Behaviour modification: An introductory textbook*. Williams and Wilkins, Baltimore.

5 Beck, A. T. and Emery, G. (1979) *Cognitive therapy of anxiety and phobic disorders*. Centre for Cognitive Therapy, Philadelphia.

6 Beck, A. T., Rush, A. J., Shaw, B. F. and Emery, G. (1979) *Cognitive therapy of depression*. Guilford Press, New York.

7 Kline, P. (1984) *Psychology and Freudian Theory: An introduction*. Methuen, London and New York.

8 Rogers, C. R. (1980) 'Client-centred psychotherapy', *Comprehensive Textbook of Psychiatry* (Freedman, Kaplan and Saddock, eds.). Williams and Wilkins, Baltimore.

9 Paolino, T. and McCrady, B. (1978) *Marriage and Marital Therapy: Psychoanalytic, behavioural and Systems Theory Perspectives*. Brunner Mazel, New York.

10 Gurman, A. and Kniskern, D. (1980) *Handbook of Family Therapy*. Brunner Mazel, New York.

11 Bancroft, J. (1983) *Human Sexuality and its Problems*. Churchill Livingstone, London and New York.

12 Duffy, W. (1975) *Sugar Blues*. Warner Books, New York.

13 A full description of the many types of alternative medicine is given in Inglis, B. and West, R. (1983) *The Alternative Health Guide*. Michael Joseph, London.

Drug Tables

Tranquillisers

Chemical name	British Trade Name	American Trade Name	Australian Trade Name	Usual maximum daily dose
alprazolam	Xanax	Xanax		3mg
bromazepam	Lexotan		Lexotan	18mg
chlordiazep-oxide*	Librium Tropium	Librium A-Poxide SK-Lygen Libritabs	Librium	100mg
clobazam†	Frisium			60mg
clorazepate dipotassium	Tranxene	Tranxene Azane	Tranxene	60mg
diazepam*	Alupram Atensine Dialar Diazemuls Evacalm Solis Stesolid Tensium Valium Valrelease	Valium	Valium Ducene Pro-Pam Lorinon	30mg
ketazolam	Anxon			60mg
lorazepam*	Ativan Almazine	Ativan	Ativan	10mg
medazepam	Nobrium		Raporan	40mg

Chemical name	British Trade Name	American Trade Name	Australian Trade Name	Usual maximum daily dose
oxazepam*	Oxanid Serenid-D Serenid Forte		Adumbran Serepax Benzotran Murelax Praxiten	180mg
prazepam	Centrax	Centrax		60mg

* Available in the UK under the NHS from 1 April 1985
† Available in the UK under the NHS for epilepsy only from 1 April 1985

Sleeping Pills

Chemical name	British Trade Name	American Trade Name	Australian Trade Name	Usual maximum nightly dose
flunitrazepam	Rohypnol		Rohypnol	2mg
flurazepam	Dalmane Felmane	Dalmane	Dalmane	30mg
loprazolam	Dormonoct			2mg
lormetazepam	Loramet Noctamid			1mg
nitrazepam*	Mogadon Nitrados Remnos Somnite Surem Unisomnia		Mogadon Dormicum	10mg
temazepam*	Euhypnos Euhypnos Forte Normison	Restoril	Euhypnos Normison	60mg
triazolam*	Halcion			250micro-grams (0.25mg)

* Available under the NHS from 1 April 1985

Common Antidepressants

Chemical name	British Trade Name	American Trade Name	Australian Trade Name	Usual maximum daily dose
amitriptyline	Tryptizol Domical Elavil Lentizol Saroten	Amitid Elavil Endep Amivil Amitril	Laroxyl Tryptanol Saroten Elavil	200mg
butriptyline	Evadyne			150mg
clomipramine	Anafranil Anafranil SR			75mg
desipramine	Pertofran	Pertofrane Norpramin	Pertofran	200mg
dothiepin	Prothiaden		Prothiaden	150mg
doxepin	Sinequan	Sinequan Adapin	Sinequan Quitaxon	300mg
imipramine	Tofranil Praminil	Janimine SK-Pramine Tofranil Antipress Imavate Presamine	Imiprin Iramil Prodepress Melipramine Somipra Tofranil	225mg
iprindole	Prondol			150mg
lofepramine	Samanil			210mg
maprotiline	Ludiomil			150mg
mianserin	Bolvidon Norval		Tolvon	200mg
nomifensine	Merital Merital AM			200mg
nortriptyline	Allegron Aventyl	Aventyl Pamelor	Allegron Nortab	100mg
protriptyline	Concordin	Vivactil	Concordin	60mg
trazodone	Molipaxin			600mg
trimipramine	Surmontil	Surmontil	Surmontil	300mg
viloxazine	Vivalan			400mg

Less Common Antidepressants

Chemical name	British Trade Name	American Trade Name	Australian Trade name	Usual maximum daily dose
flupenthixol	Fluanxol			3mg
iproniazid	Marsilid		Marsilid	150mg
isocarboxazid	Marplan	Marplan	Marplan	30mg
phenelzine	Nardil	Nardil	Nardil	60mg
tofenacin	Elamol			240mg
tranylcypromine	Parnate	Parnate	Parnate	30mg
tryptophan	Optimax Optimax WV Pacitron			6g

Note
Although these tables of tranquillisers and sleeping pills do indicate British trade names, it is important to remember that prescriptions under the NHS from 1 April 1985 onwards will not give the trade name but the chemical one. Drugs listed under the column headed 'Chemical name' and bearing asterisks are the *only* ones which are able to be prescribed by name on the NHS. This ruling does not apply to the antidepressant drugs on pages 159–60.